CONQUERING
INCONTINENCE

Peter Dornan has been a physiotherapist in the fields of sporting injuries and manipulative therapy for the past 35 years, working with many international sporting teams, including the Queensland rugby team, the Wallabies and the Kangaroos. Peter has also been an Olympic advisor and Commonwealth Games physiotherapist. He is a fellow of Sports Medicine Australia, and has written two successful books on sporting injuries. In 2000 he was awarded the Commemorative Australian Sports Medal for achievement in sport.

In recent years Peter's interests have turned to men's health and the treatment of incontinence patients, and in 2000 he was awarded the Duncan Travelling Fellowship to study aspects of prostate cancer in the United States. In 2002 Peter was appointed as a Member of the General Division of the Order of Australia (AM).

Peter Dornan has published two previous books with Allen & Unwin, *The Silent Men* and *Nicky Barr, An Australian Air Ace*.

Peter has been married to Dimity, a speech pathologist, for more than 35 years, and they have two children, Melissa and Roderick.

CONQUERING
INCONTINENCE

A new and physical approach
to a freer lifestyle

Peter Dornan

ALLEN&UNWIN

First published in 2003

Allen & Unwin
83 Alexander Street
Crows Nest NSW 2065
Australia
Phone: (61 2) 8425 0100
Fax: (61 2) 9906 2218
Email: info@allenandunwin.com
Web: www.allenandunwin.com

National Library of Australia
Cataloguing-in-Publication entry:

Dornan, Peter, 1943–.
    Conquering incontinence: a new and physical approach
    to a freer lifestyle.

    Bibliography.
    Includes index.
    ISBN 1 74114 144 3.

    1. Urinating disorders. 2. Urinary incontinence—Treatment.
    I. Title.

616.62

Set in 12/14.5 pt Granjon by Midland Typesetters, Maryborough, Victoria
Printed by McPherson's Printing Group, Australia

10 9 8 7 6 5 4 3 2 1

I dedicate this book to my wife, Dimity Dornan. Besides being my primary support system, my tireless cheer squad leader when problems seemed insurmountable, and my critical life editor and coach, she is my inspiration and muse, the well-spring of all creativity.

Never give in, never give in—never—in nothing, great or small, large or petty—never give in except convictions of honour and good sense.
—Winston Churchill

Contents

Figures

Acknowledgments

A book of this nature relies heavily on the support of not only members of the medical profession, but also on the many sufferers, survivors and patients who have shared their problems and experiences with me.

I would particularly like to acknowledge the role of my friend and urologist, Dr Les Thompson, for his consistent encouragement, countenance and direction over the last seven years. I am also extremely grateful to the many other urologists, oncologists and doctors who have assisted me to further my understanding in this area.

I am indebted to the members of the Queensland branch of the Continence and Women's Health Special Group of the Australian Physiotherapy Association. There were many special people within this group who assisted me with advice and ready back-up. In this regard, I would like to give particular thanks to Dr Ruth Sapsford for her continuing championship. I would also like to pay tribute to physiotherapists Prue Ryan and Jackie Lander.

I am also obliged to the dedicated staff at the Queensland Cancer Fund who have encouraged and assisted me in so many marvellous ways. I would especially like to mention psychologist Suzanne Steginga for her perspicacity and sound judgment relating to psycho-social concerns.

On matters relating to mountaineering, I would like to give particular thanks to Drs Alan Frost and John Taske, as well as to Jim and Marianne Drapes of Peregrine Travel.

A special accolade also goes to my dedicated office manager, Carol Jackson, whose patience and assistance in both typing and compiling the many drafts of this manuscript have been invaluable.

Finally, I wish also to express my gratitude to the many caring friends I have met both internationally and locally, especially through the now wide network of the Australian Prostate Cancer Foundation. In particular, I am obliged to the members from my own affiliated Brisbane Prostate Cancer Support Group. The collective courage, humility and support demonstrated by individual members continues to inspire me.

I will never underestimate the power of the human spirit.

Peter Dornan
Brisbane 2003

Glossary

after-dribble annoying dribble that exists after urination
   has finished
anti-cholinergic agents drugs which block the contraction of the bladder muscles
anticipatory reflex the reflex which prepares postural
   muscles for movement
benign prostatic hyperplasia enlarged prostate
biofeedback/electrical stimulation a system to assist pelvic
   floor muscle training
bladder container which stores urine
bladder augmentation a surgical procedure to treat severe
   bladder instability
bladder sphincter weakness weakness of the cuff (sphincter) which prevents leakage from the bladder
bladder training techniques a program to train the
   bladder to void normally
bulbospongiosus muscle muscle on the penis which surrounds urethra
bulking injection injection around the bladder neck with
   bulking material
collateral circulation an alternative circulatory system

continence to contain urine in the bladder

cystoscope an instrument for viewing inside the urethra and bladder

depression cycle a regular drop in mood

detrusor the muscular coating of the bladder

dorsal vein of the penis complex a large collection of veins surrounding the prostate

fast-twitch muscle fibres muscle fibres which specialise in speed movements

feed-forward mechanism see *anticipatory reflex*

glans penis head of the penis

internal sphincter strong ring of muscle which forms a cuff around the urethra

ischaemia loss of blood in a tissue, restricting arterial inflow

kidneys glandular organs intended for the secretion of urine

levator ani collective term for the three pelvic floor muscles

local circulation the blood supply around a specific area, e.g. prostate

magnetic therapy magnetic current utilised for therapy, e.g. pain relief, muscle contraction

micturition the act of passing urine

'nerve-sparing' operation surgery to remove the prostate and spare the nerves around it

neural reflex circuitry nerve network mediated by reflexes and command centres

neuropraxia compression or stretching of a nerve

obliques abdominal muscles aligned obliquely

Onuf's nucleus   located in the sacral cord, it controls the complexities of continence and the evacuation of the bladder and bowel

over-active bladder   sensitive bladder muscle that reacts inappropriately to stimuli

pelvic floor muscle exercises   a set of exercises designed for continence management

pelvic floor muscles   layers of muscle which form the pelvic floor

pons, or midbrain   joins various segments of the brain

prostate   walnut-shaped gland of the male reproductive system

prostatectomy   removal of the prostate

PSA test   a blood test to determine the health of the prostate

rectal sphincter   a cuff of muscle around the rectum

rotator muscle groups   abdominal muscles which rotate the spine

sacral cord   the section of spinal cord which is situated in the sacrum

slow-twitch muscle fibres   muscle fibres which specialise in endurance functions, e.g. posture

suburethral sling   a surgical procedure designed to lift the urethra

transversus abdominis muscle   an abdominal muscle important to trunk stability

tricyclic antidepressants   pharmacologic agents reported to be useful for treating urge incontinence

unstable bladder   over-sensitive to inappropriate stimuli, causing urge incontinence

ureters   the tubes draining urine from the kidneys to the bladder

urethra   the tube draining urine from the bladder to the outside

urethral sphincter   strong ring of muscle which forms a tight cuff around the urethra

urge incontinence   an inability to defer urination

urinary diversion   a surgical procedure to assist in treating urge incontinence

urinary sphincter   a strong muscular ring around the urethra

urination centre   the command centre for urination. It controls continence and voiding and is situated in the pons

voiding   the act of emptying the bladder

Introduction

Urinary incontinence is perhaps the most widespread yet least known and understood affliction facing people today. Incontinence is the inability to properly control the passing of urine, so that it is passed at inappropriate times or inappropriate places. Incontinence can be an intense personal disaster for those afflicted, as well as being costly for individuals, institutions and governments in human and economic terms if it is not effectively treated and managed.

This book is written primarily as a self-help program for those suffering from incontinence—particularly stress incontinence, which is defined later in the book. It will also be a useful reference tool for doctors, physiotherapists, urology nurses and all those who have a special interest in incontinence or who are affected by it.

Life may not always be the party you wished for, but while you are here you may as well dance.

—Anon

When I was diagnosed with prostate cancer at the age of 52, after a routine blood *(PSA) test*, the shock was enormous.

At the time, I didn't even know what my prostate was—or, for that matter, what it did. And I certainly took the functioning of my urinary system for granted. As well, as a health professional—a physiotherapist—I had followed a lifestyle for the last twenty years which the gurus had promised would significantly lessen the risk of cardiac disease and cancer. However, it proved to be not completely so.

To add to the shock, virtually any invasive treatment I could undertake had the potential of being nasty. To me, at the time, surgery (radical *prostatectomy*) seemed to offer the best chance for survival. At this stage, some seven years later, it certainly appears to have achieved that—something for which I am decidedly grateful.

However, after the prostatectomy in February 1996, I was left severely incontinent, to the extent where I was filling six incontinence pads a day during the first three months. As this rate of leakage was not improving, and I found that it was seriously impacting on my lifestyle as well as my professional career, emotional health, exercise activity and sex life, I became fairly despondent. In desperation, I sought out some physiotherapy colleagues.

They taught me how to execute standard *pelvic floor muscle exercises*, which I performed aggressively and with enormous motivation. Over the next two weeks, this action stemmed the flow to between one and two pads a day, a far more manageable situation. By the end of twelve months, I had controlled the loss to about a dozen leakages a day.

While this was now more acceptable and manageable in terms of my lifestyle, I found I had acquired a distressing legacy which had developed from the original traumatic period of the diagnosis and the time immediately following the prostate surgery. During this early stage, when I initially considered I might be permanently incontinent and might have to give up my life as a physiotherapist, as well as many other activities which enhanced my quality of life, I developed a *depression cycle*.

Just one leakage would remind me of the desperation associated with the trauma of the diagnosis, the horrendous decision-making process and the now obvious psycho-social legacies resulting from my choice of treatment. I repeatedly challenged myself with the useless questions: 'Did I choose correctly? Should I have undergone this surgery?'

Several specialists whom I consulted agreed that whatever urinary function I had at the end of the first year, in terms of 'stress incontinence', was probably what I would have forever.

The frustration, anger—and, indeed, often rage—I felt at my situation led me to form the first Prostate Cancer Support Group in Queensland. From this, I hoped to find some answers to assist both me and the many others I soon found who were fellow sufferers. The Brisbane Prostate Cancer Support Group is now one of the largest support groups in the country, with over 600 men and their partners on the mailing list.

My incontinence remained at this same level (about a dozen leakages a day) for approximately four years. At this stage, I was awarded a special travelling fellowship from the Queensland Cancer Fund. This enabled me to travel to the United States in 2000, to attend various clinics to develop my understanding of incontinence. (By now, I had been treating other men, but only to this same limited degree of success.)

During a period of research at the Cleveland Clinic, one specialist I interviewed gave me an almost throw-away line, one which I eagerly picked up on. He (and eventually others) speculated that the long-term neural deficiency which could lead to *bladder sphincter* (the muscle, or cuff, which controls the urine outlet) *weakness* (a partial and possible cause of stress incontinence) may be attributed to severe damage to the blood vessels supplying these nerves, causing an inadequate flow of blood (*ischaemia*).

Embracing my background in sports medicine, with its inherent assertive ethos, and by applying my experience and training in exercise physiology, I considered it may be possible, with intensive conditioning, to influence the *local circulation* and maybe introduce a *collateral circulation* to this area, that is, to stimulate the growth of an alternative circulatory system. (For instance, consistent training has been shown to cause the iliac artery of an athlete to adapt from an average of 6 millimetres wide to 12 millimetres.) The specialist at the Cleveland Clinic agreed the concept was feasible.

During this time, I was also becoming aware of recent research into the relationship between posture, *neural reflex circuitry* and bladder control. In the context of my situation, this information led me to focus and concentrate on retraining what is known as the *anticipatory reflex*.

The anticipatory reflex is triggered when the central nervous system (brain or spine) receives a message to perform a major postural change. For example, when we are required to extend the arm, as in executing a hand-shake, a split-second before the message is relayed to the muscles which move the arm forward, this anticipatory reflex (or *feed-forward mechanism*) sends a message to command the relevant major postural muscles to contract. This action effectively increases intra-abdominal pressure in preparation for a change in trunk stability.

In particular, the diaphragm, the abdominals and pelvic floor muscles all contract simultaneously in an effort to control pelvic and trunk stability, thus countering the forward momentum generated by the moving arm (and therefore preventing the body from potentially falling over).

If there has been any significant damage to elements of the neural network which supplies the integrated contraction of these muscles (from surgery, trauma or disease of any kind), and as a result it renders the pelvic floor muscles slow to contract and therefore suffer a degree of incoordination, the increased intra-abdominal pressure may lead to some leakage.

My plan, therefore, was to try to retrain this reflex cycle by introducing speed and agility movements aimed at 'jiggling' and stimulating structures involved with this cycle.

So, on my return to Brisbane some four-and-a-half years after surgery (with my incontinence still maintaining a steady dozen leakages a day), I increased my usual 30-minute, four-times-a-week jog to about 50 minutes, eventually building up to running over rough mountain pathways. In an effort to retrain and improve the reflex cycle, I also started zig-zagging, bounding over rocks and generally added exercises that created sudden posture changes.

After three months following this routine, my incontinence dropped from a dozen down to about three leakages a day. Initially, I suspected the improvement may have been attributed to a strengthening of the bladder sphincter, as a result of the stimulus of the overload work program. However, as fate would have it, I then damaged my knee and could not run for three months. But after the three-month lay off, I was delighted to find that I could maintain this low level of incontinence.

This led me to hypothesise that I may well have introduced a collateral circulation. If I had merely increased the neuromuscular strength of the sphincter, I believe this would have been lost with the marked decrease in exercise.

The next improvement came from applying some research which came from the Physiotherapy Department of the University of Queensland. This new evidence reinforced the empirical observation that there was a clear functional connection between the pelvic floor muscles and the muscles controlling the abdominal and pelvic cavity. It was shown that voluntary abdominal muscle activity, particularly of the transversus abdominis and oblique muscles, is associated with pelvic floor activity.

Functionally, this makes sense. When lifting a heavy weight, for instance, the diaphragm, abdominals and pelvic floor muscles all contract simultaneously to create an increased intra-abdominal pressure, thus channelling the force off the spine.

So I altered my normal abdominal exercise routine to deliberately incorporate and co-activate the pelvic floor muscles. Lying on the floor, with my knees bent up,

I would brace and flatten my abdominals to ensure maximum contraction of the rotators and transversus abdominal muscle groups. Concurrently, I would then pull up (contract) my pelvic floor muscles and execute an abdominal 'crunch' routine, building up to 400 reps a day. A wit once accused me of living the philosophy 'If a thing's worthwhile doing, it's worthwhile overdoing'. In this instance, it proved to be the key!

After another few months, the leakage diminished to maybe a few drops every few days. This was something I could definitely live with! But the best result was that it also broke the depression cycle.

The Final Test:
Mt Kilimanjaro, Tanzania, February 2003

It is exactly seven years now since I was first diagnosed and treated for prostate cancer. The experience has been compelling, exhausting, frustrating and, in some instances, quite claustrophobic, yet in many ways it has been enlightening, and even liberating. However, seven years on I feel the need for a sense of closure—something I hope to achieve by climbing Mt Kilimanjaro in Africa.

Why climb a mountain to prove anything? Most people would consider the exercise to be irrational.

Perhaps, on one level, I see some symbolism of the uphill climb cancer survivors must face and overcome. On another level it is, of course, an opportunity to measure oneself.

I turn 60 in March. The climb, I realise, will probably test my physical and emotional capacities to the limit. I take the challenge of ageing seriously, and acknowledge the need to live comfortably within certain limitations. However, I also believe that a man's reach should exceed his grasp; I believe it is imperative to keep striving, to keep fuelling the drive to survive, to struggle, to do better, to create and be fulfilled. So I need to keep challenging myself from all aspects—physically as much as intellectually.

Finally, of course, the main reason I'm undergoing this climb is to test my program for treating stress incontinence. If I can climb Kilimanjaro, I will hopefully prove its effectiveness.

Mt Kilimanjaro is the tallest mountain in Africa. It lies close to the equator, yet snow, ice and glaciers are found on its highest slopes. Soaring to the impressive altitude of 5895 metres (nudging 20 000 feet), it provides incredible views of hundreds of square kilometres of surrounding countryside—thousands of metres below—as well as of the surrounding mountain peaks, valleys and glaciers.

The 60-kilometre climb to the summit takes you through a number of distinctly different climatic and vege-tation zones—from beautiful rainforest, which is often hot and stifling, to moorland, alpine desert and, finally, glaciers, ice and snow, where the temperature can drop as low as minus 20°C.

I am ready for the test. My injured knee has been arthroscopically treated, and I have been training for some time. I feel as ready as I can be.

I am happy to report that now, some seven days later, I have successfully breeched the summit. There were times when I seriously questioned why the blazes was I up there in the rarefied atmosphere, slogging through snow, mud and scree in minus 10°C temperatures, and being pelted with rain, hail and snow. But in the end I have tested my physical and emotional capabilities almost to the limit and come out on top. It took five days of seven to eight hours walking a day to reach the summit. In some respects, it was even more challenging coming down as the knees and Achilles tendons were unrelentingly, eccentrically pounded over two more hard days.

However, more importantly I believe the climb well and truly proved the effectiveness of my incontinence treatment program as, over the course of the week, the only time I lost any fluid was once during the first two days when I suddenly lifted my backpack onto my shoulders. By the third day, however, particularly after the urological neural reflexes possibly had a chance to be strongly trained and integrated with the reflex systems controlling both feet, the hands working two walking poles, plus the abdominals, diaphragm and pelvic floor muscles, my continence control moved to a new level—I have rarely had a significant leakage since.

Even though the climb had its moments of stress and discomfort, there were many rewarding incidents which more than made up for the temporary hardships. Let me take you through some highlights of the fifth, and to me the longest, day—the attempt at the summit.

After four days of hard climbing and trekking, at 4545 metres we were instructed to have four hours sleep. Our guide would then wake us at 10.30 pm, allow us a cup of tea, then lead us in darkness on a seven-hour walk directly to the summit, in time for sunrise. We would then return to camp and have a break before continuing downhill on a five-hour walk to our next camp, below the height where we would be most likely to develop serious altitude sickness— a total of fifteen hours walking for the day.

We always knew this day would be hard and there were some anxious moments as we tried to sleep. We were all well aware that this period is the stage when most deaths occur, and 80 per cent of climbers are forced down before reaching the summit. Sleep was difficult as these thoughts weighed heavily on my mind. In particular, it concerned me that, should altitude sickness symptoms become so severe as to cause serious cerebral or pulmonary oedema, skilled medical help was at least two days swift hiking from here.

Another more pertinent concern for me related to incontinence. Should I lose any urine while in this potentially freezing climate, the chance of suffering frostbite to sensitive anatomy seemed a realistic possibility. A troubling thought.

A snowfall had rolled in off the summit during the short night and the temperature had dropped to freezing. Wind snapped at our tents, whipping and cracking them and our anxiety increased. But joyously, when we were woken at 10.30 pm for our cup of tea, we were greeted by a beautiful full moon and a landscape bathed in white, interspersed with black rock.

As we climbed, the scene took on an eerie, almost surreal atmosphere. Down below on the African plain, lights from the local villages twinkled back at us, as in a fairyland. Over to our left and below us, a violent thunderstorm built up, crashing its loud warning as lightning flashed and darted around the sky. It was really quite marvellous.

By about 3 am, the moon slipped behind the mountain, and the scene suddenly became chillingly dark. We switched on our torches and continued trudging uphill, fighting against snow, rock and mud, and very unstable scree. Breathing became difficult now, and every footstep became a major task. At our last camp I needed one or two breaths per footstep. Now, close to the summit, I needed five breaths to sustain one footstep.

At this stage, around the cone a certain unspoken drama was being played out as at least a dozen international teams converged towards the summit. Trails of light were seen dotting the steep gradient as climbers desperately searching for oxygen and energy called on their every resource to commit to the summit. Sadly, some lights were seen to turn back, the effort too great.

I was now needing seven lungfuls of air per step, and though exhausted, I still felt in control and knew I had some energy in reserve. Finally, I reached the top at about 6.30 am, accompanied by an unsurpassed sense of relief and achievement.

What a tremendous way to see Africa—from its roof! From its highest point, peering out into the mists of distance, and indeed time, it was not hard to imagine the teeming animals on the plains far below waking as the first rays of the sun ignited the ancient landscape. After all, this is where life on earth began. The words of the song 'Morning has Broken' must have been inspired by such an emotion . . . 'Like the first morning'.

I have been encouraged by my own experience to use this routine on incontinence patients referred to me as a result of prostatectomies. The results have been remarkably rewarding, demonstrating a consistently high degree of success. The patients themselves have been impressed with the results, and I have every confidence that, with some reservations, the routine will also assist many females diagnosed with stress incontinence.

At this stage, some seven years after treatment, I consider my triumph to be fairly complete.

My thoughts go back to a passage I was reminded of during my darkest hours. A friend, ethicist Noel Preston, suggested I keep looking for 'the gift in all this'. He related that the writer John O'Donohue had once stated: 'Often the most wonderful gifts arrive in shabby packaging.' From the comfort of this moment and the state of my present good health, nothing I say should camouflage just how shabby that packaging was. However, over time, the gifts have revealed themselves.

As I moved from loss to life, from woundedness to wholeness, and from longing to acceptance, Noel revealed another O'Donohue insight: as the body ages, the soul gains in richness, becoming deeper and stronger. But the greatest gift to me was the renewed awareness that my need for family and friends was far greater than any other drive, need or ambition.

The following pages outline the philosophy and simple steps needed to follow the program, which have been the outcome of these insights.

Outline of the book

To achieve maximum benefit from the program outlined in this book, it is important to spend time understanding some of the fundamental workings of the bladder, particularly in relation to its functions of *voiding* and *continence*—that is, expelling and containing urine. As such, it is necessary to learn a little about the anatomy and physiology of the structures that make up the lower urinary tract, as well as being aware of what constitutes normal bladder function. These two subjects are covered in Part I, setting the scene for the rest of the book.

Part II defines urinary incontinence, then discusses the various possible causes of this condition before examining the standard treatment options. This helps to create a firm setting to understand the rationale for the new approach, which is outlined in detail in Part III.

Part IV focuses on the legacies of prostate cancer, as well as dealing with the 'demons' of the depression cycle and the issue of erectile dysfunction.

Part I
Anatomy and physiology:

The bladder and the lower urinary tract

1

How it all works

The urinary system: An overview

The urinary system is composed of four major parts: the kidneys, the ureters, the bladder and the urethra.

The *urethra* extends from the neck of the bladder and, in the female, exits the body in front of the vaginal opening; in the male, it passes through the prostate gland and exits at the end of the penis (see Figure 1.1).

The *kidneys*, situated in the flank area under the ribs on either side of the body, filter water and waste material from the blood to form urine. The kidney excretes what the body no longer needs, and channels this urine through a long narrow tube, the ureter, to where it collects in the bladder.

The *bladder* really is a reservoir, or storage chamber. Its walls are composed of special cells which become thick and muscular when empty. As the bladder fills, the walls stretch and become thinner; full capacity is reached at around 500 millilitres. As the bladder reaches about 40 per cent capacity—roughly 200 millilitres—an initial message is triggered telling the brain that it is time to empty. At this stage, the brain can then make a conscious decision to either hold or release the contents. As the bladder becomes fuller, the messages increase in frequency to the extent that a strong urge to pass urine—even to the point of pain—may be experienced (the crossed leg stage). Some people (about 10 per cent of the population) have bladders that over-respond to these messages and don't allow the bladder muscle to relax in order to accommodate a reasonable quantity of urine. These bladders are referred to as *unstable* or *over-active*.

For urine to be released through the urethra, the *urinary sphincter* must relax. (The sphincter is a strong ring of muscle which forms a tight cuff around the urethra.) After voiding, the sphincter then contracts (or tightens) again. The muscle, often called the *internal sphincter*, is comprised mainly of *slow-twitch muscle fibres*. This enables the sphincter to stay continually working—that is, it allows the sphincter to maintain continence by ensuring urethral closure for long periods.

This muscle is generally compromised by radical prostatectomy and takes time to recover. It fatigues early during the recovery process—which is why most leakage often occurs during the afternoon, or later in the day.

The pelvic floor

The floor of the pelvis is made up of layers of muscle and other tissues. There are three muscles which form the pelvic floor and they are collectively called the *levator ani*,

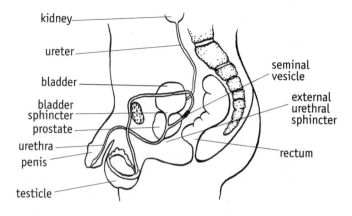

Figure 1.1a   Male pelvic organs

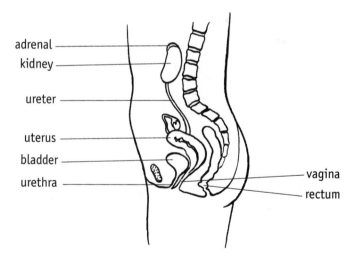

Figure 1.1b   Female pelvic organs

which means simply 'to lift the anus'. These pelvic floor muscles (see Figure 1.2) stretch like a hammock from the tailbone at the back to the pubic bone at the front. Their main function is to act like a diaphragm to support the contents of the pelvis, particularly the bladder and bowel, and the uterus in the female. The pelvic floor muscles also surround the urethra, vagina and rectum as they pass through to the exterior. In the context of this book, the pelvic floor muscles play an important role in bladder and bowel control by contributing to both the *rectal sphincter* and the *urethral sphincter* mechanisms, thus providing bladder neck support and supplementary urethral closure.

Generally, the pelvic floor muscles are made up of about two-thirds slow-twitch muscle fibres, which allow them (like the sphincters) to stay continuously tonic (working), underlying their role in supporting the pelvic organs. The specific pelvic floor muscles around the urethral sphincter

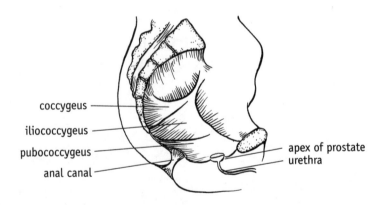

coccygeus

iliococcygeus

pubococcygeus

anal canal

apex of prostate
urethra

Figure 1.2   Pelvic floor muscles

are a mixture of *fast-twitch* and slow-twitch muscle fibres that raise urethral closure pressure during periods of increased intra-abdominal pressure (such as during sustained lifting). The presence of fast-twitch fibres means that the pelvic floor muscles can also quickly and reflexly contract to support the urethral sphincter while we are performing sudden heavy lifting, coughing or the like.

The prostate

The *prostate* is a small, walnut-shaped gland of the male reproductive system. It is located at the neck of the bladder like a collar surrounding the urethra as it descends from the bladder (see Figure 1.1).

The gland produces fluid which provides one of the constituents of semen and becomes part of the ejaculate. This fluid has a role in sperm mobility. During ejaculation, as the sperm enters the urethra, the bladder neck contracts (tightens) to propel the ejaculate down the urethra.

The prostate gradually enlarges with age, creating the potential to cause what is known as *benign prostatic hyperplasia* (BPH), or 'enlarged prostate'. Depending on the degree of enlargement, this can constrict the urethra, causing a degree of obstruction and slowing the urine outflow.

There is a large neurovascular bundle between the prostate capsule and the rectum. These nerves relay messages from various centres to both the bladder and the penis. Damage or interference to these nerves during surgery can interfere with both continence and potency.

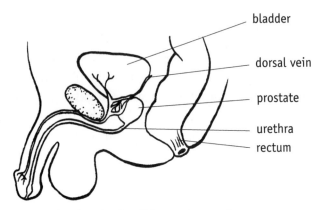

bladder

dorsal vein

prostate

urethra
rectum

Figure 1.3   The dorsal vein of the penis complex

There is also a large collection of veins surrounding the prostate. The veins are called the *dorsal vein of the penis complex*. When removing the prostate, surgeons have to be careful not to injure these veins, as they carry a large amount of blood.

Abdominal muscles

For this program to be effective, it is essential that the role of the abdominal muscles and the diaphragm in the management of incontinence is understood.

Recent research has reinforced the empirical observation of the strong link between abdominal muscle activity and pelvic floor muscle activity. There is evidence that *transversus abdominis*, the diaphragm and the pelvic floor muscles coactivate to form an enclosed abdominal cavity in a response designed to control spinal stability (Hodges,

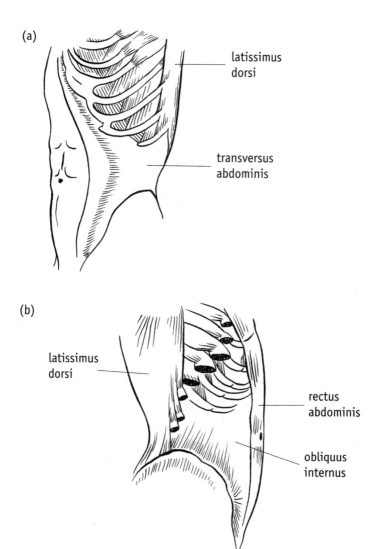

Figure 1.4   The abdominal muscles highlighting (a) *transversus abdominis*, (b) the rotators—*obliquus internus* and (c) *obliquus externus* (see p. 24)

(c)

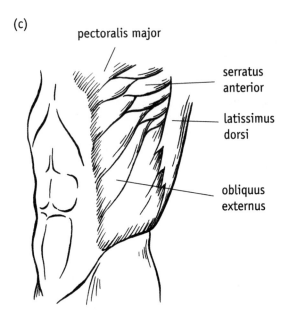

pectoralis major

serratus anterior

latissimus dorsi

obliquus externus

1999) (Figure 1.4). Further contraction of *obliquus externus*, *obliquus internus* and *transversus abdominis* muscles (Figure 1.4) has been shown to occur automatically during a maximum pelvic floor muscle contraction (Sapsford et al., 2001). In fact, in another study (Sapsford and Hodges, 2001) it was found that increasing strength of abdominal muscle activity was associated with increasing activation of pelvic floor muscles.

This program places a strong emphasis on developing fit abdominal muscles in order to help overload and increase the fitness of the pelvic floor muscles.

In relation to reflex circuitry, and in particular the

anticipatory reflex (discussed in the Introduction), experimental evidence has shown that, when arm movement is performed, the onset of *transversus abdominis* activity precedes that of the deltoid muscle (the shoulder muscle which moves the arm forward) by approximately 30 milliseconds (Hodges and Richardson, 1997).

Further, testing of the diaphragm indicates that shortening of the diaphragm precedes the onset of shoulder movement, providing further confirmation of the mechanical efficiency of the feed-forward activation of the diaphragm (McKenzie et al., 1994).

Nerve supply to the urinary system

The nerve supply of the lower urinary system is complicated. However, some understanding of its functioning is necessary.

There are thirteen reflexes which control bladder voiding and continence. These reflexes are mediated through at least seven command centres, ranging from centres in the brain and spinal cord to nerve centres in the bladder wall, as well as the urethral sphincter and pelvic floor muscles, in a coordinated manner.

Central to efficient bladder control in the male is the internal sphincter of the bladder (see Figure 1.1a) (there is no internal sphincter in females). This is controlled by the autonomic nervous system (which controls the body's involuntary movements). All neural sensory fibres from the pelvic region ultimately feed into what is known as *Onuf's nucleus* in the *sacral cord*, which then coordinates and controls the complexities of continence and evacuation of the bladder and bowel.

To further complicate things, the autonomic nervous system is divided into the sympathetic and parasympathetic divisions, or trunks (see Figure 1.5). The sympathetic division allows bladder storage, while the parasympathetic produces a sustained bladder contraction for emptying. When the genitalia are stimulated, impulses reach the spinal erection centre situated in these trunks (the nerves carrying these impulses enter and exit the

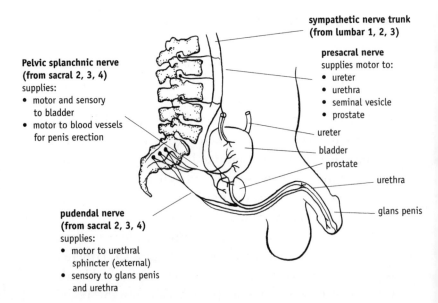

Pelvic splanchnic nerve (from sacral 2, 3, 4) supplies:
• motor and sensory to bladder
• motor to blood vessels for penis erection

sympathetic nerve trunk (from lumbar 1, 2, 3)

presacral nerve supplies motor to:
• ureter
• urethra
• seminal vesicle
• prostate

ureter

bladder

prostate

urethra

glans penis

pudendal nerve (from sacral 2, 3, 4) supplies:
• motor to urethral sphincter (external)
• sensory to glans penis and urethra

Figure 1.5   Nerve supply to the bladder and urethra

spine at the sacrum outlets, S2 to S4, and thoracic and lumbar vertebrae outlets, T10 to L2), causing the penis to become erect. The pelvic floor muscles (including the anal and urethral external sphincter) are supplied by the pudendal nerves.

With all these factors in mind, it is not difficult to visualise how any interference applied to this sensitive neural network, from childbirth (in the female), surgery or other trauma (to either male or female), could have a marked effect on continence control. (In the case of the male, it can also contribute to erectile dysfunction.)

Coupled with the natural anxiety involved with both the loss of bladder control and sexual function, this situation could very quickly escalate into a syndrome involving serious psycho-social legacies if it is not addressed as quickly as possible.

Normal bladder function

As discussed in Chapter 1, normal bladder capacity is about 500 millilitres. It takes an average of 15–30 minutes for a glass of water to be passed through the system to reach the bladder if the patient is well hydrated. When the bladder fills to about 200 millilitres, the first signal to void is registered in the brain. This normal urge can be suppressed until the bladder fills to about 400–500 millilitres. At this time, the desire is felt again and voiding occurs. If the situation is not convenient, then the bladder can easily defer and eventually accommodate up to 700–800 millilitres.

The normal frequency of voiding is between four and six times a day, and perhaps once a night. This varies with fluid intake, activity and ambient temperature, and can increase to around six to eight times a day in the elderly.

As the bladder enlarges (at about 200 millilitres), stretch receptors in the bladder walls discharge a message to a part of the midbrain (the *pons*—known as the *micturition* or *urination centre*), which has both facilitary and inhibitory capabilities. This message is then relayed on to the cerebral cortex, leading to conscious awareness, so that one feels the urge to void at this point.

If one chooses not to void, reflex bladder contractions subside within a minute or so, and urine continues to accumulate. After about 200–300 millilitres more has collected, voiding generally occurs. On the other hand, at the appropriate time, if one wishes to void, the cortex sends a message via the pudendal and pelvic nerves causing the pelvic floor muscles and urethral sphincter to relax. A few seconds later, another message relayed via the parasympathetic nerves initiates bladder muscle contraction, therefore allowing urine to flow.

Urine should then flow in a steady continuous stream without discomfort. Unless the abdominal wall and pelvic floor muscles are relaxed for voiding, flow will be slow, intermittent and incomplete. There should be no hesitancy or strain; there should be minimal residual in the bladder or urethra; and no *after-dribble* should occur. If there is some after-dribble, it is usually due to weakness of the muscle which surrounds the urethra (the *bulbospongiosus muscle*). This is very common in males over the age of 40 and has nothing to do with the prostate. It can be helped by specific exercises.

In order to remain continent, the following are necessary:

- a bladder which is able to remain relaxed while filling, and able to contract to completely empty on voiding;
- a strong sphincter mechanism;
- a pelvic floor strong enough to support the sphincter mechanism;
- an intact neural network system; and
- a healthy vascular system to supply nerves and muscles.

Erectile dysfunction and orgasm

In relation to erectile dysfunction—a well-recognised side-effect of prostate cancer as well as its treatment—many factors are involved which are beyond the scope of this book. However, it is useful to know that, from a diagnostic point of view, they may be classified as psychogenic, vasculogenic, neurogenic, endocrinologic, diabetic, drug-related, trauma-related and poor pelvic musculature. In relation to this book, if there is a chance that the cause is purely neurogenic, vascular or caused by weak pelvic floor muscles, this program may be helpful in working towards a recovery.

The other associated and useful piece of information concerns male orgasms. The experience of orgasm is independent of sympathetic and parasympathetic activity, which is often compromised during radical prostate surgery, but it does require an intact pudendal nerve, which is rarely involved during prostate surgery (see Figure 1.5) (Mamberti-Dias et al., 1999). So, although radical prostatectomies may interfere with erections, orgasms are nearly always preserved. Of further interest, a transurethral resection of the prostate (TURP)—a treatment for enlarged or benign prostate hyperplasia (BPH)—will interfere with neither erections nor orgasms.

Part II
Incontinence:

Causes and treatments

2

What causes incontinence?

Defining incontinence

Urinary incontinence is defined as the complaint of any involuntary leakage of urine (International Continence Society, 2002).

Urinary incontinence can be a major health problem. Because of the social stigma often associated with it, incontinence has traditionally been under-reported, and many patients are hesitant to discuss the problem with their physician and other health care professionals.

Even though the condition was previously almost exclusively seen in women and older men, in this era of increased detection of prostate cancer in men and the intervention of radical prostatectomy for treatment, post-prostatectomy incontinence (PPI) is also now becoming an increasing problem. All incontinence is troublesome, but PPI is particularly disturbing because it generally occurs in men who had normal continence immediately before surgery. The same could be said for women who develop incontinence after childbirth or surgery.

There are basically four types of incontinence:

- stress incontinence;
- urge incontinence;
- overflow incontinence; and
- mixed incontinence.

Stress incontinence

This occurs when any movement or action that increases pressure in the abdominal cavity results in urine leakage. The condition manifests itself with such activities as coughing, sneezing, laughing, heel impact upon walking or running, changing posture (sitting to standing), sexual activity or passing wind. Because there is often fluid loss caused from impact during sport, sufferers often adopt a more sedentary lifestyle, which can eventually lead to further health issues.

Urge incontinence

When the urge to 'go to the bathroom' is so great you cannot 'hold it', it is referred to as urge incontinence. The bladder muscle (*detrusor*) contracts in spasm so strongly it squeezes fluid out. The leakage is accompanied, or immediately preceded, by urgency.

(Motor) urge incontinence can also be known as 'unstable or overactive bladder', and can be associated with 'frequency' (frequent voiding). As such, loss of control can also be triggered by, for example, the sound of running water or approaching the front door lock (on the way to the bathroom). Sensory causes can be from urinary infections, stones and cancer.

I have a patient who has urge incontinence and will not leave the house for fear of not being able to make it to the next toilet. Her condition is of such concern to her that she has memorised the locations of all the local public toilets in her area. The urge can be triggered without warning when she hears a steady high frequency sound such as whistling, upon which she will simply 'lose it'.

Overflow incontinence

Also called false incontinence, overflow incontinence is when the bladder never drains completely because either the urethra and/or bladder neck is obstructed or the bladder muscle (detrusor) contracts very poorly. The urine subsequently builds up behind the sphincter and overflows like water over the top of a full drain.

Mixed incontinence

Commonly, components of all these types of incontinence, such as stress and urge incontinence, can occur together. Often, however, one symptom (either stress or urge) is generally more bothersome to the patient than another. Identifying the most annoying symptom is important when targeting diagnostic and therapeutic interventions.

Incontinence is not a disease; nor is it a natural part of growing old. Incontinence is a symptom or side-effect of other health concerns, which can range from faecal impaction to brain tumour.

Common causes of urinary incontinence

There are a number of common causes of urinary incontinence, including:

- urinary tract infection;
- idiopathic detrusor (bladder wall) over-activity (instability);
- bladder outlet obstruction;
- faecal impaction causing straining;
- being overweight;
- heavy lifting;
- pelvic floor muscle weakness;
- giving birth;
- stroke;
- dementia;
- diabetes;
- chronic cough;
- lack of general fitness; and
- impaired mobility.

Many other rarer causes also exist, many of them leading to weakness of the pelvic floor muscles and resulting in urinary incontinence.

Incontinence in females

As well as any of the other causes mentioned above, incontinence in females often occurs as a result of pregnancy and childbirth (vaginal delivery), vaginal prolapse and oestrogen deficiency.

In cases where childbirth leads to incontinence, it is important to avoid surgical therapy postpartum (after the birth) until the condition does not resolve. Behavioural intervention is the primary choice of treatment for most women. Observations suggest it is vaginal delivery rather than pregnancy that causes pudendal nerve damage leading to incontinence.

Another common cause of incontinence in females is urinary tract infections, with the patient presenting symptoms of frequency and urgency. The immediate form of treatment is generally antimicrobial therapy.

Incontinence in males

As well as many of the factors mentioned above in 'common causes', incontinence in men can be a result of prostate enlargement, as well as a consistent side-effect of most invasive treatments of prostate cancer, particularly prostatectomy and radiation therapy. Incontinence can be caused by damage to the neuromuscular bundles around the prostate. It may also result from devascularisation and fibrosis (scarring), or loss of elasticity, of the sphincter mechanism—or both. Among men who undergo radical prostatectomy surgery, the condition is temporary and resolves itself over time in 80–90 per cent of cases.

Most men are dry enough after three months not to have to wear a pad. However, a small percentage may have continuing leakage requiring pads. After two years, surgeons perceive that up to 35 per cent of men will be left with stress incontinence and less than 5 per cent experience severe incontinence.

3

Conventional treatments for stress incontinence

The three major categories of treatment for stress incontinence are behavioural, pharmacologic and surgical. As a general rule, the first choice should be the least invasive treatment appropriate for the patient, which offers the fewest potential adverse effects.

For most forms of urinary incontinence, especially stress incontinence, behavioural modification techniques meet these requirements.

Behavioural modification

Pelvic floor muscle exercises

Pelvic floor muscle exercises were first described to treat female stress incontinence by gynaecologist Dr Kegel (thus the name Kegel exercises), in 1951. There is emerging evidence that they also clearly help men with post-prostatectomy incontinence (Moul, 1998). For instance, a recent controlled trial supports the intervention of physiotherapy treatment for men with post-prostatectomy urinary incontinence (Van Kampen et al., 2000). These findings are supported by other experimental evidence (Moul et al., 1998; Meaglia et al., 1990). Even in men who subsequently regain full control, experience and clinical evidence suggest that properly performed pelvic floor muscle exercises allow more rapid return of control—or, at the least, that they lessen the eventual degree of stress incontinence (see Chapter 4).

External penile clamp

The first penile clamp was invented over 60 years ago to control the dripping associated with gonorrhea. Invented by a Dr Cunningham, it was called the Cunningham clamp. Gonorrhea has since been treated more effectively with sulphur drugs, but men have since used the clamp to control incontinence. However, few have accepted its use because of the associated discomfort.

A commercial product called the Squeezer™ Klip is more comfortable, as two longitudinal bumps on the top arm apply downward pressure as they straddle critical blood vessels. This device can be worn for long periods of time, giving complete control.

For more details on the Squeezer™ Klip, go to the product's website: <www.GeezerSqueezer.com>.

Biofeedback/electrical stimulation

These techniques help patients who have trouble isolating the pelvic floor muscles or who are very weak in this area.

The patient must be kept very relaxed and, with the aid of a monitor screen, can be trained so that he or she localises the pelvic floor muscles only. (Electrodes are inserted in the rectum in the male, and in the vagina in the female with one placed on the perineum.) The technique does increase functional bladder capacity and improves the tone, contractility and efficiency of the pelvic floor muscles. Its main drawback is that it only appears to stimulate the fast-twitch muscle fibres and not the important slow-twitch endurance fibres. Overall, it has not been shown to be any more effective than voluntarily performing simple pelvic floor muscle exercises.

Clinical trials are currently being conducted on a new non-invasive treatment called *magnetic therapy*. This involves a therapeutic magnetic field that initiates contractions of the pelvic floor muscles. The patient sits in a special chair, fully clothed, and the machine does the work. However, only time will tell whether it is any more effective than voluntary contractions (the device is not cheap— at US$24 000).

Modifications to diet and fluid intake

It is increasingly being recognised that dietary factors can exacerbate urinary incontinence. Alcoholic beverages, cola, milk, coffee, tea, caffeine, citrus products, tomato, highly spiced foods, sugar, honey and chocolate may all irritate the bladder and lead to detrusor muscle instability.

It is also important to maintain adequate hydration. Specialists recommend drinking 2 litres of fluid a day—

that is, eight glasses of water. Recent evidence has shown it is not necessary to be hung up on drinking just straight water—other beverages are fine. However, depending on what you drink, it may be necessary to keep an eye on the kilojoules. Soft drinks and sports drinks can be high in sugar content—which can quickly go to your gut.

Further, if you find that soft drinks and caffeine don't irritate your bladder, the *Journal of the American College of Nutrition* recently featured a small study showing that when men drank caffeinated beverages, they were as well hydrated as when they downed an equal amount of water (*Men's Health*, 2002).

Bladder training

The goal is to progressively extend intervals between voidings, typically to a period of three to four hours (see Chapter 5, which discusses urge incontinence).

Pharmacological intervention

There are many drugs available which can assist stress and urge incontinence. Because of potential side-effects, however, the risk-to-benefit ratios are often difficult to gauge. The patient should consult carefully with his/her doctor to ascertain which particular drug may be most helpful in each individual case.

For instance, in cases of moderate or severe urge incontinence involving detrusor muscle over-activity, it has been shown that drug therapy—such as *anti-cholinergic agents*—can reduce the instability, but does not usually eliminate it, so it should be used in conjunction with pelvic floor muscle exercises and bladder training techniques (refer to Chapter 5). In fact, these drugs have quite significant side-effects, especially in the elderly, so they should only be used temporarily as an adjunct to the other treatments.

Further, for treatment of stress incontinence, it has been shown that alpha-adrenergic agonist drugs can stimulate both striated and smooth muscle tone, which can increase urethral resistance. However, side-effects such as anxiety, insomnia, agitation, respiratory difficulty, sweating, cardioarrythmia and hypertension can limit the drugs' appropriateness.

Surgical intervention

The objectives of surgical treatment of incontinence depend on the specific causes and diagnosis. A given patient may have more than one cause for their condition. While it is not the role of this book to discuss every procedure available, it can be useful to know that surgical procedures may be useful for several purposes:

- to increase outlet resistance of the urethra to relieve stress incontinence;
- to decrease detrusor instability to help correct urge incontinence; and
- to remove outlet obstruction in order to correct

overflow incontinence or to reverse detrusor instability that is secondary to the outlet obstruction.

Surgery may only be recommended for treatment of stress incontinence as a first-line treatment for appropriately selected patients if other non-surgical therapies are not effective.

Bulking injections

Periurethral injections of the bladder neck area with bulking material are supported by clinical trials as a first-line surgical treatment. It is a minimally invasive technique performed under local anaethesia. It can be effective for both males and females, although women who are found to have a coexisting hypermobility problem of the urethra should have that assessed and addressed first. The aim with the latter condition is to improve the support of the sphincter unit without anything obstructing it.

For both sexes, a *cystoscope* is inserted inside the urethra and up into the bladder, through which bovine (cow) collagen or autologous (from self) fat is injected into the bladder neck. This has the effect of narrowing or closing the opening, although this opening retains the ability to expand normally upon voluntary urination (see Figure 3.1).

The patient may need three or four treatments for maximum effect, although experience and follow-up have shown that this treatment is often limited, as the collagen or fat is often flattened out or absorbed into the local tissues. The effectiveness often only lasts for three months to a year.

Surgeons are now trialling a synthetic substance called macroplastic which appears not to absorb into the system as readily as collagen. This is a formula of collagen particles which have been immersed in an oil solution substance to give solidarity, and which coagulates in the tissues. Trials using a cross-linked bovine collagen substance have demonstrated reasonable effectiveness at two years.

For males, it appears to work best post-prostatectomy rather than for post-radiation treatment, where there appears to be too much scarring for it to be effective.

The literature does not support the use of bulking agents in men with severe post-prostatectomy incontinence. They seem to work best for mild stress incontinence (less than two sanitary pads a day).

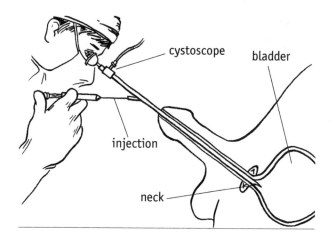

Figure 3.1   Bulking injections

Suburethral slings

'Slings' have been used in women for many years and are performed mainly for treatment of complicated incontinence, although they are often recommended for sphincter deficiencies as a first-line treatment. The various sling procedures all involve placing a sling, made of either autologous (self) or heterologous material, under the urethrovesical junction and anchoring it behind the pubic bone or to abdominal structures, or both. The success and complication rates vary with individuals.

The Stamey sling for men and other sling procedures are undergoing clinical trials in several United States hospitals. The operation involves the placement of three non-stretchable tubes across the urethra to act as 'bolsters' to the bladder neck and prevent leakage. It is a minimally invasive technique, cheaper than an artificial sphincter and so far has had impressive short-term results.

Artificial urinary sphincter

For severe incontinence (more than three pads a day), it may be worthwhile considering the artificial sphincter, although it is advisable to wait at least two years after behavioural and pharmacologic intervention have been tried.

The artificial sphincter is a surgically implanted device requiring a general anaesthetic. It consists of a cuff placed around the urethra or bladder neck which can be inflated manually to prevent urine leakage.

The artificial sphincter has been shown to have good

results for 95 per cent of men, although there has been considerable bad press given to complications and side-effects. These are involved mainly with mechanical problems and malfunctions, erosion of the cuff into the urethra and pump erosion. For more information on the artificial sphincter visit the AMS Sphincter 800 information guide at the American Medical Systems website at <www.visitams.com/pdf/21600045.pdf>.

Part III
Behavioural intervention:

A new and physical approach

4

A new approach: Taking control

Nothing in the world can take the place of persistence.
—Calvin Coolidge

Taking a new approach

This program focuses on expanding the philosophy involved with *behavioural intervention*, particularly in relation to pelvic floor activity. It is based on the role of the pelvic floor in providing bladder neck support and supplementing the required pressure to close the urethra.

The prime focus is to develop a highly efficient (super-fit) neuromuscular and vascular system which controls and supplies all the structures that form the pelvic and abdominal cavities, including the pelvic floor muscles. Further, as mentioned earlier, as there are seven command centres which control bladder voiding and continence, it is essential that a specific intense system of exercise be undertaken to improve all reflex circuitry relating to this control. In this regard, it is also important to retrain neuromuscular elements which relate to the anticipatory reflex (see the Introduction and Chapter 1).

For incontinence involving nerve damage—and I refer particularly here to the *'nerve-sparing' operation* for men who have undergone a radical prostatectomy—any nerve damage in this instance should be *a neuropraxia* (compression or stretching of the nerve), and the pathway should reactivate within nine months to two years. However, recent evidence (Apell, 1999) suggests that the main damage during surgery is probably to the blood vessels supplying the nerves, and this may be one cause of long-term neural deficiency. In view of this speculation, the longer-term purpose of this program is to stimulate and functionally retrain the efficiency of the local vascular system to the extent that a collateral circulation may be introduced. (This is not unreasonable. An average man can increase the width of his iliac artery from 6 millimetres to 12 millimetres through dedicated aerobic training.)

Further, during the process, elements of the muscular and neural system will also be dynamically retrained, hopefully leading to a more normal bladder control situation.

The program aims to achieve these goals at four levels:

1   to gain control, strength, power, endurance and speed of muscle contraction of the *pelvic floor muscles*;
2   to dynamically and functionally retrain and integrate the *pelvic floor muscles* with the *abdominal muscles*;
3   to dynamically and functionally retrain components of the *reflex circuitry* involved with continence to enhance the continence mechanism; and

4   to aerobically condition elements of the *local vascular system* supplying neural and other structures in the pelvic region.

Note that for males being treated post-radical prostatectomy, because of the risk of developing an inguinal/incisional hernia, the abdominal exercise component (level 2) should be commenced with some care. It would be advisable to wait at least two to three months after surgery before heavy abdominal exercises are undertaken.

Similarly, women need to be aware that there are many different pathologies which can cause stress incontinence. Women will also need to be careful for some months after uro-genital and/or abdominal surgery, limiting any resistance exercises to below 15 kilograms. If there is any concern, a doctor should be consulted before this program is commenced.

The program

Level 1: Pelvic floor muscle exercises

The following pelvic floor muscle exercises are standard but specific exercises routinely prescribed for continence management. There are three exercises in this level of the program. Before actually starting the routine, it is important to understand that we are trying to train the muscles for both improved muscle endurance (i.e. the slow-twitch muscle fibre response) and for speed of muscle contraction (i.e. improved function of the fast-twitch muscle fibre response). This dual attack is to allow the muscles to provide stronger and more enduring bladder neck and sphincter support, such as when standing, as well as eventually to provide a faster reflex contraction, such as is required during a sneeze, cough, etc.

Keep in mind the fact that the pelvic floor muscles are comprised predominantly of slow-twitch or endurance fibres. Therefore, these pelvic floor contractions need to be practised at a *slow* rate and then a *fast* rate. The following is a suggested routine.

- *Slow:* Contractions should be sustained at maximum intensity for five seconds (or longer).
  Routine: Contract—hold—two-three-four-five—relax (repeat five times).
- *Fast:* Contractions should be performed as quickly as possible, ensuring each one is a full contraction.
  Routine: Contract–relax, contract–relax (repeat for five contractions).

Be aware that the muscles will tire quickly in the early stages. Wait for them to completely relax before you 'pull them on again' (in other words contract them). It may take some seconds for them to recover completely before the next 'pull on' is possible. *Always* wait for complete recovery before 'pulling on' again.

While performing the following exercises, focus on the pelvic floor muscles, not on the other muscles around the pelvis.

Exercise 1

Imagine you are at a party and you are trying desperately to prevent passing wind (from the bowel). Tighten and contract the muscles around the anal sphincter. The sensation will be similar to that as if you are drawing your anus up into your bowel. Learn to be aware of what it feels like to tighten (or pull on) the muscles and then relax them.

Exercise 2

Imagine you have a full bladder and you are passing urine. Now envisage trying to stop the flow midstream by tightening the muscles underneath the penis or vagina. Then relax the muscles. For a test, it's worthwhile trying this exercise initially while actually passing urine; this will give you some idea of how much strength and control you have over this muscle. If you can't stop the stream, note the performance level and test it again in a week's time.

Exercise 3

In the early stages, this exercise is often performed more efficiently lying down. With the knees bent up and the feet placed on the floor, locate the perineal area (the perineum) between your anus and scrotum or vagina. Imagine you are holding a red hot needle which you aim at this region. By contracting the pelvic floor muscles, pull your perineum away from the 'needle', back inside the body. To a male, it will feel like you are drawing your testicles up into your lower abdominal region.

Exercise 4
When you have mastered the above three exercises individually, the next exercise is to contract *all* the muscles involved in the above three exercises *together*, as if you are trying desperately not to lose any urinary or faecal matter. As soon as you can achieve an efficient contraction of all these muscles together, you no longer need to perform them individually again. In the future, you will need only ever do exercise 4.

Regularity
While learning the exercises, a reasonable goal in the early stages is to try to complete the full program twice a day. As you achieve control, add one or two more sessions. Do not set unrealistic goals—for instance, attempting up to ten sessions a day may lead to boredom and probable non-compliance. In fact, it is the intensity rather than the frequency of work that is important. The bottom line, however, is that *you must never give up: you must persist.*

Once you can efficiently do exercise 4, you are ready to incorporate the exercises from level 2.

Warning: If an exercise causes pain, either during or after its performance, cease exercising and seek advice from a physiotherapist experienced in treating these conditions.

Level 2: Integration of pelvic floor muscle activity with abdominal muscle activity

Recent research has shown a strong link between abdominal muscle activity and pelvic floor muscle activity. For instance, during heavy lifting it has been shown that the abdominal muscles, the pelvic floor muscles and the diaphragm all contract simultaneously. This has the effect of increasing the intra-abdominal pressure, thus converting the trunk into a 'rigid cylinder'. The main advantage of this is to increase the mechanical stability of the spine, thus allowing stress to be shunted down the legs instead of through the spine. Further, as stated in Chapter 1, researchers at the University of Queensland have shown that the abdominal muscles—especially *obliquus externus*, *obliquus internus* and *transversus abdominis*—contract automatically during a maximal pelvic floor contraction.

So, once the patient has gained control of the pelvic floor muscles (using level 1 exercises), the next step is to coordinate these with all other muscles involved with pelvic and trunk stability, especially the abdominals.

To train this integrated mechanism effectively, it is important to ensure that, during exercise, the abdominal muscles are deliberately contracted at the same time as the pelvic floor muscles (that is, while performing the fourth pelvic floor exercise).

There are many variations and levels of abdominal exercises. The patient's fitness status will determine which degree of difficulty is chosen. Generally, I prefer to start with the basic and traditional 'crunch' exercise. It is one most individuals are familiar with, and can easily be overloaded to gain improvement. But no matter what level you commence at, it is important to isolate the *obliques* (or *rotator muscle groups*) to ensure full abdominal muscle efficiency.

Instructions

- Lie on your back with your knees bent and your feet flat on the floor.
- To isolate the abdominal rotator muscles, place your fingers on the large muscles located just in front of your hip bones, then cough. You should feel them stiffen or contract. These are the muscles we are trying to work.
- To make them work functionally, imagine someone is about to deal a blow to your lower abdomen. Brace against this by drawing your lower abdomen and navel down towards your backbone and the floor. This position is the starting position for all abdominal exercises—that is, with all abdominal muscles braced hard and flat as if you are wearing a corset (or brace).
- The abdominals are now contracted and ready to work.
- Coactivate—'pull on'—your pelvic floor muscles (the fourth level 1 exercise) at the same time.
- With your hands behind your head in order to protect your neck, and with your neck muscles relaxed, use your abdominal muscles to raise your trunk, shoulders and head as in a half sit-up (or crunch), while still sustaining the pelvic floor contractions (see Figure 4.1).
- Then lower the head, shoulders and trunk.
- To more deliberately work the rotators, as you sit-up or crunch, aim and move the right elbow towards the left knee and then vice-versa (see Figure 4.2).

If you are grossly unfit, start with three repetitions, and do not try to lift your head and shoulders very far. To progress, the magic increment for overload is about 10–15 per cent. Be very patient—you may need to stay on one level of repetitions for days (or even weeks or months).

Abdominal exercises

- Bent leg sit-ups (crunches).
- Sit up, keeping abdominals flat.
- Brace abdominals (flatten into bed) and pull on pelvic floor muscles.

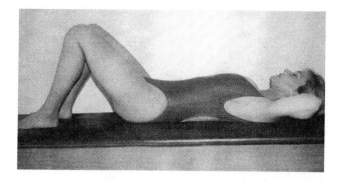

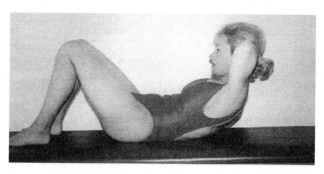

Figure 4.1   Basic crunch exercises

As you get fitter, build up to the bicycle manoeuvre. Begin with your hands behind your head. Then use a bike pedalling motion to crunch your left knee to your right elbow; then alternate sides (see Figure 4.3).

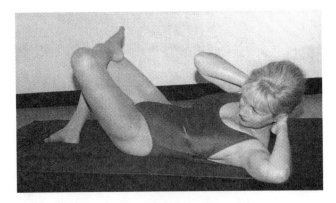

Figure 4.2   Obliques (rotators) and transversus

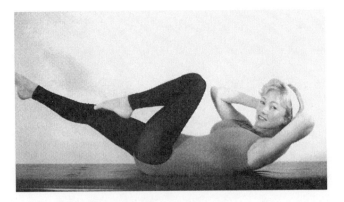

Figure 4.3   Cycling and trunk rotation

Increasing your fitness

As you adapt to a particular fitness level, try to increase the intensity of your exercise by 10–15 per cent, to eventually accumulate a session tally of all combined abdominal and pelvic floor muscle exercises which reaches at least 200 repetitions. However, it's important that the increase be gradual. You may find it necessary to stay at the one level for three weeks before you are fit enough to move on. (Elle McPherson does 400 a day—it would be nice to secretly aim for that!)

You can increase the resistance and difficulty of the routines by choosing exercises that generate a greater percentage of activity in the abdominal muscles. For instance, the bicycle manoeuvre generates almost two-and-a-half times more activity than the basic crunch. Some intermediary activities include the long-arm crunch (a basic crunch with your arms extended above, and in line with, your head) and the vertical leg-crunch (a basic crunch with your legs raised to 90 degrees and knees slightly bent. Your legs should remain still as you crunch).

Level 3: Retraining the reflex circuitry mechanism

This routine is aimed at dynamically and functionally retraining components of the reflex circuitry mechanism involved with incontinence to enhance the continence mechanism.

It involves activities which train the pelvic floor muscles around the urethra while carrying out functional activities.

Initially, the aim is to contract the pelvic floor muscles during walking, building through to jogging, then up to hard running, eventually pounding over hills and uneven tracks.

The intention here is to 'joggle' the internal neural systems about in an attempt to stimulate and retrain the bladder reflex circuitry, particularly the anticipatory reflex (see Chapter 1).

Begin the routine by contracting (pulling on) the pelvic floor muscles at the beginning of a gentle walk. Aim to hold the contraction as long as possible, although in the early stages they may tire quickly after walking only a few metres or for a few seconds. Let them relax and recover. Pull them back on again—they may 'fade' again even quicker than the first time. Do not worry. You may even leak—put up with it. After they have recovered, pull them on again. Continue in this pattern until the pelvic floor muscles are exhausted. With training, they will eventually hold on for longer.

As the muscles adapt, it is important to overload by increasing the degree of difficulty of the terrain and therefore heel impact, building up to hard, uneven surfaces.

Do not be impatient with this routine. It may take several weeks—even many months—before significant improvement in bladder control is noticed.

Second, you need to train yourself to contract the pelvic floor muscles while performing other dynamic activities which increase abdominal pressure. For instance, when you move from sitting to standing, quickly pull the pelvic floor muscles on in preparation.

Similarly, before lifting, pull the pelvic floor muscles on

(correct lifting technique also requires the abdominal muscles to be braced at the same time). Likewise, when coughing or sneezing, contract the pelvic floor muscles as quickly as possible before the cough occurs.

In fact, for any activity or function in which an increase in abdominal pressure has forced you to leak, you should practise contracting the pelvic floor muscles just before that particular activity.

These activities should be performed as exercises, with the idea being to shorten the reflex time needed to contract the pelvic floor muscles before the activity, so that eventually the pelvic floor muscles, abdominals and diaphragm will automatically coordinate and co-contract in preparation for the activity.

Level 4: Conditioning the vascular system

This routine is designed to aerobically condition elements of the local vascular system supplying neural and other structures of the pelvic region. The aim is to create an enhanced or collateral vascular system supplying any damaged nerves in the urogenital area.

Ultimately, this involves an overload aerobic training program, such as cycling or running. As with the level 3 routine, the pelvic floor muscles are co-contracted while performing the endurance activity, with the aim of stimulating the need for an increased blood supply to all the local structures in the urogenital area (including neural structures), and therefore regenerating a new or collateral circulation.

Of course, levels 3 and 4 can both be attained concurrently by creatively utilising the same activities—walking, to jogging, to running, and so on.

Pilot study: Testing the program

In support of this more aggressive philosophy of managing incontinence, I commenced a pilot study to test the concept.

The program was instituted on fourteen consecutive post-prostatectomy patients who had developed incontinence as a side-effect of surgery. The average age of the men was 63.5 years, and they were first instructed on the program at a mean of two months post-surgery. At this stage, the patients needed, on average, 3.5 sanitary pads a day. Each patient's progress was monitored at monthly intervals.

The results are set out in the Appendix on page 99.

Discussion of pilot project

After an average of six months on the program, ten of the men (73 per cent) were found to be completely dry, while three patients (21 per cent) still had a small amount of leakage (a few drops daily). One man was unable to continue with the program as he developed diverticulitis and a post-operative hernia. The remaining thirteen patients were delighted with the result.

The results of this pilot study do appear promising, and there are indications that further research would be worthwhile.

5

Urge incontinence and bladder training

Patience is bitter, but its fruit is sweet.
—Aristotle

I have a friend who is a businessman and a member of a number of boards, which involves regular meetings and long hours of discussion. Two years ago he had a procedure to relieve pressure on his urethra as a result of an enlarged prostate. This had the effect of irritating the bladder muscle, to the extent that he would regularly receive an inappropriate message to go to the toilet. He would immediately attend to the urge and would be disappointed to note that his bladder was nowhere near full.

He began to combat this by not drinking water before meetings, which didn't assist either the urge or his general health. He became so anxious that he might not make it to the toilet in time that he positioned himself closest to the door. Eventually he would feel the urge to go simply by having a glass of water sitting nearby on the table. In time, even tinkle sounds, such as those made by a glass, car keys or an ashtray, would trigger his urge. Life became very stressful for him.

Urge incontinence is described as an inability to defer urination, usually accompanied by a strong urge or 'need to go'—in other words, an inadequate warning to reach the toilet before voiding commences. Patients simply can't 'hold on'; the urge to urinate is excessively strong and the episode may well result in leakage—even uncontrollable flooding—before the toilet is reached.

This 'need to go' can be influenced by rainy days and heightened by cold. It can also readily be triggered by the sound of running water. Commonly, the problem can develop into a sensitive conditioned response, to the point where a simple action such as placing the keys in the front door of the house in anticipation of going inside to access the toilet can stimulate the urge.

Frequently, urge incontinence occurs when the circuitry to the brain has become confused. This can occur to the extent that it cannot tell whether the bladder is actually 'full', or whether it is receiving a false—and urgent—message that it needs to void.

With awareness, however, the patient can be taught the difference between the sensation of a full bladder and that of urge incontinence. The feeling of a full bladder occurs in the lower abdomen just above the pelvic bone, whereas urge incontinence is felt around the urethra—around the base of the pelvis for men, and deep inside the vagina for women. Once you are aware of the difference, you can learn to beat urge incontinence.

Urge incontinence reflects a wide range of causes, including what is known as an *unstable bladder*. This relates to the *detrusor muscle* (bladder wall muscle) reacting to any number of inappropriate stimuli and over-contracting, setting off the sensation of needing to 'go'. Many local irritative bladder conditions can set it off—menopause, bladder stones, urinary tract infections and tumours. It can also be associated with neurologic conditions such as stroke, spinal cord lesions and multiple sclerosis. In males—particularly the elderly—an enlarged prostate can also trigger off urge incontinence. As well, men who have had prostatectomies often are left with a legacy of a combination of stress and urge incontinence. Obviously, these conditions need to be initially diagnosed by a doctor and any medical aspect appropriately treated.

Urge incontinence can even be an end process of habits begun as a child—practices such as going to the toilet 'just in case', before a car ride, going to school or before an event, can set up an anxiety reaction where the bladder becomes improperly trained. Instead of waiting for a natural urge to warn the child that it is time to consider going to the toilet, a synthetic 'need' is implanted over the bladder circuitry, confusing the normal system. In time, many different stimuli can begin to trigger the need to 'go'.

Whatever the cause, however, most cases of urge incontinence develop because the bladder has taken over command of the urinary process—it has over-ridden the other command and reflex centres that normally orchestrate what should be a smooth, automatic function.

The importance of the pelvic floor muscles to urinary control has already been established. If any component of the reflex system involving the pelvic floor muscles, including weakness of the muscles, is compromised, it can have the effect of relaying an inappropriate message to the brain, causing it to lose the ability to be aware of when it is 'full'.

For this and other reasons, the central focus of management of urge incontinence should be to gain strong control of the pelvic floor muscles with the intention of regaining command of the inherent bladder and brain circuitry.

Management options

Pharmacological interventions

Anti-cholinergic medications are often used, as they block contraction of the muscles of the unstable bladder. Side-effects include a dry mouth, drowsiness, constipation and vision accommodation difficulties.

Tricyclic antidepressants should be reserved for carefully evaluated patients, as they are known to produce many adverse side-effects, particularly cardiac problems.

Behavioural techniques

As already mentioned, the best strategy to manage urge incontinence is to pursue a very disciplined exercise program aimed at putting the pelvic floor muscles back in charge. The idea is to suppress the over-active bladder by inhibiting detrusor muscle contraction by a strong voluntary contraction of the pelvic floor muscles at the same time as the urge to void is experienced. Second, this should be backed up by clearly understanding and practising *bladder training techniques* (see below).

Pelvic floor muscle exercises

Quite simply, the main aim of this program is to try to create enough stimuli, by any means, to over-ride the flawed messages going to the bladder which are telling it to void early. One of the most effective means of achieving this is by developing a 'super-fit' pelvic floor musculature so that it can 'beat', or 'over-ride', the other messages going to the bladder—that is, to resist or inhibit the sensation of urgency. The other effect of developing powerful pelvic floor muscles, of course, is that it can physically prevent leakage by compressing the urethra.

The pelvic floor program should be followed as described in Chapter 4. Particular importance should be directed at the role of the abdominal muscles to enhance pelvic floor muscle strength and endurance. Like any fitness training schedule, it may take some weeks—even months—for this to be effective. After all, not only are the pelvic floor muscles trying to physically prevent urine leakage, as well as attempting to regain neural command, they also often have to over-ride and reprogram a long-term, well-entrenched habitual cycle.

Bladder training

People who suffer under the 'tyranny' of urge incontinence often tend to take evasive action in advance. They frequently choose to 'go' before they have to—just in case: before car trips, shopping trips, classes, functions, and so on. Very quickly, their bladder 'trains' *them*. Ultimately, they lose the ability to 'hold on' at all, as their effective bladder capacity steadily shrinks. Eventually, the bladder becomes so sensitive, or unstable, that it fires voiding messages to the brain at the slightest possible stimulus. It never gets 'full'.

The basic concept of bladder training—or, as it is often termed, bladder 'retraining'—consists of three main principles. The program requires the patient to:

1   resist the sensation of urgency;
2   postpone voiding; and
3   urinate according to a timetable, rather than a urinary urge.

These tactics help distend the bladder by increasing fluid loads and assist to create longer intervals between voids.

It is therefore important to *increase* fluid intake so the bladder can distend and be a better reservoir. Most patients suffering from urge incontinence tend to *restrict* fluids, which is completely the wrong thing to do.

Initially, the goal is simply to extend the time between the first sensation of an 'urge' and when the patient just *has* to void. If the patient can 'hang on' for, say, 30 seconds extra, then this is the target to be beaten next time. The following time, the patient may then 'hang on' for a longer interval before voiding, eventually building up to a normal two or three hours.

The essential step is to reach the toilet early, and then to undress *before* the urine begins to flow. Unless a person can do this, they have no chance of deferring.

Obviously, the stronger and fitter the capabilities of the pelvic floor muscles, the longer the duration of hold.

There is, of course, an element of mind-play in this concept, as well as sheer physical strength. A certain amount of resolve, determination and discipline is needed to withstand the compulsion of a powerful 'knee-crossing' urge. One element needed for victory will be the development of a philosophy of 'not letting it win'. With patience, persistence and training, it is possible to steadily overcome this urge.

Other deferment measures can also be used. Such techniques as sitting on a rolled-up towel or applying direct hand pressure to the perineal area in an effort to aid the effect of the pelvic floor muscles to close the urethra can be helpful. Even sitting on the arm of an appropriate chair will have a useful effect.

If your mind is strong enough, you can also utilise *distracting* thoughts to divert attention from the urge—think about a favourite holiday, mental puzzle or something challenging and pleasing. This takes some concentration, but if you can sustain the distracting effort even for 30 seconds, the urge can often melt away.

As already mentioned, the other important aspect of bladder training is ensuring adequate fluid intake. Never cut back on your fluids, as this will add to the negative cycle by decreasing the ability of the bladder to expand effectively. As mentioned in Chapter 3, try to maintain a regular 2 litres a day, which will keep the bladder under regular stress so that it can be retrained. Also, keep in mind that it takes about fifteen minutes for a glass of water to move through a well-hydrated person's system into the bladder. This knowledge can help in planning a suitable 'training' time—one where you can give full concentration to overcoming the urge.

The bottom line to maintaining a healthy bladder, in this context, is that you should only go to the toilet when the bladder is full.

Be aware that some cases of urge incontinence may be more complicated than this, and not all people will respond to this program. It is important to consult a urologist under these circumstances.

Let's go back to my friend, the businessman, whom I introduced at the beginning of the chapter. As an individual he is very strong-willed, and was determined to overcome his bladder problem. A former athlete, the idea of a committed and disciplined exercise program appealed to him and suited his temperament.

Over several weeks he built up to 600 sit-ups per exercise session, combined with an hour walk up a small hill in his local park five times a week. At the same time, he built up his fluid intake with the idea of challenging and training the bladder to accept more fluids. As his fitness improved, he concentrated fiercely to overcome his urge. Six months later, he had not only succeeded in controlling most of his urge incontinence, but he had also recommenced practising a healthy lifestyle.

Finally, surgical procedures such as *urinary diversion* and *bladder augmentation* can be recommended for those patients with intractable, severe bladder instability or poor bladder compliance that is unresponsive to all other therapies.

Part IV
Cancer and incontinence:

The psychological and social effects

6

Dealing with the demons: Cancer, depression and beyond

If you don't laugh at trouble, you won't have anything to laugh at when you are old.

—Ed Howe

The psycho-social legacies of prostate cancer

When a man is diagnosed with prostate cancer, it is not just his life that is threatened. Besides dealing with the shock of the trauma from the diagnosis, there is a realisation that practically any medical treatment has the potential to impact upon other important body functions. Surgery and radiation both have the potential to compromise bladder control and sex life, while radiation can also damage other local anatomical features, especially the bowel. Further, hormone therapy (anti-androgen therapy) can also produce various side-effects—loss of libido and erectile dysfunction, osteoporosis, cardiovascular problems, hot flushes and many more.

The implications of these 'psycho-social legacies' often don't appear too important in the early days of the cancer diagnosis, as the urgent focus is on trying to survive. However, once this crisis subsides, most men hope to resume their previous lifestyle. This is when they realise that their quality of life may have been greatly affected, as they grapple with the realities of the side-effects—a situation often creating great concern.

Research has shown that many of these men can quickly slip into periods of reactive depression, a phenomenon many of them may not have experienced previously. This can occur when there is an overwhelming feeling of loss or sadness; life has slipped out of their control and they can't immediately find clear answers. In reality, of course, the loss is something that they have traded for their life, yet it is often difficult to accept and cope with this actuality.

It is important to recognise this 'down' period if it does occur. In most instances—as with any grief process—with time and understanding the patient will work through it into acceptance. However, if denied or undisclosed, he may quickly move into more serious clinical depression, a diagnosis needing medical intervention.

This chapter and the next may assist men through these early periods. This chapter offers a general strategy for understanding and coping with depression and flashbacks related to the diagnosis period. The next deals with the sensitive subject of erectile dysfunction and its impact.

Rise of the demons

When confronted with a stressful situation, our natural reaction is basic fear and/or anger. Whether facing an enemy in the jungle, being involved in a hold-up or receiving a cancer diagnosis, the human body reacts in a definite, clear-cut and well-defined electro-chemical response pattern.

Even witnessing a nasty traffic accident can illicit the same series of reactions—your senses become acute, your vision narrows, your heartbeat races, your hands become cold and clammy, your armpits perspire, your breathing becomes serious and concentrated, and your body assumes a readiness posture, with all skeletal muscles (especially in the neck and back) becoming taut and prepared.

As well as eliciting the above reactions, and regardless of the degree of trauma, such incidents also have the potential to produce a long-lasting psychological response. If not addressed or understood, over time a phenomenon occurs which is often interpreted and labelled by the affected individual as 'demons'. These 'demons'—memories of the experience (or flashbacks)—can be as devastating and debilitating as any physical legacy, possessing the ability to return and haunt an individual over a long period, unless they are treated.

Within a few seconds of the impact of the original stressful event, the body's automatic protective reaction is to trigger a chain of events which stimulates the nervous system. The main effect is to release adrenalin and other hormones into the system to control the situation (as described above). During this initial encounter, the brain is often overwhelmed with information which it cannot immediately process.

The cerebral cortex and neural networks, in an attempt to deal with the new (and mostly negative) information, effectively move into overload mode. In medical terms, the brain becomes traumatised or inflamed. A great deal of this scrambled information involves the presentation and selection of different choices—presumably with different outcomes—which could have been considered during those early dramatic moments. In reality, the majority of these choices would most likely have been unreasonable, risky or even impossible.

At a later date, when the confusion settles, often a simple and sometimes seemingly unrelated incident can 'trigger' the mind to relive the traumatic aspects of the event. At this stage, these bad memories, or 'demons', emerge and can trouble the individual, often challenging the person with the prospect that he/she may have made the wrong decision.

For instance, consider the case of the bank teller involved in a hold-up. In those terrifying first few seconds when the would-be robber points the gun at him (or her), the immediate choice is to use common sense and hand over the money. However, other more heroic and generally unreasonable choices, complete with a different perceived outcome, compete for that first reaction: 'Should I punch the evil-doer? Should I push the alert button under the desk? Should I scream, faint or go for my own gun?' No matter what choice the teller originally opted for, these thoughts—or 'demons'—can return to haunt him/her, particularly if the event led to the acquisition of a physical injury or disablement, thus setting up a long-lasting 'trigger'.

This process becomes easier to understand when you review some of the latest research into the human brain. Basically, a brain cell may receive incoming messages from hundreds of thousands of connecting points every second. Acting like a vast telephone exchange, the cell will instantaneously compute the sum data of all incoming information and will redirect it along the appropriate path.

As a given message, or thought—or, in this case, a relived memory—is passed from brain cell to brain cell, a biochemical/electromagnetic pathway is established. Each of these neuronal pathways is known as a *memory trace*.

Every time you have a thought, the biochemical/electromagnetic resistance along the pathway carrying that thought is reduced. The more times the message travels that path, the less resistance there will be until, after many repetitions, the messages have developed a wide, smooth track that requires little clearing. Simply, the more the brain repeats patterns of thought, the less resistance there is to them. Significantly, the more times a 'trigger event' happens, the more likely it is to happen again.

This concept, of course, is very useful—and indeed desirable—for learning things, particularly good things. Unfortunately, it is also quite simple to learn negative things, as with the bank teller's unlucky experience.

Prostate cancer's particular demons

This scenario is not too different from the situation of a man diagnosed with prostate cancer. Initially, the emergency is that if the patient does not act, he may well die.

The alternatives for treatment are not always pleasant or easy, since virtually any medical choice comes with a high risk of acquiring a legacy that can seriously affect the patient's quality of life. He finds he is indeed between a rock and a hard place.

Once he has chosen a treatment plan, the eventual undesirable side-effects of treatment—along with other triggers—can release the bad memories related to the traumatic diagnostic process. Such symptoms as faecal and/or urinary incontinence, failed sexual performance (as a direct result of surgery or radiation), stress fractures, hot flushes, memory lapses, cardiovascular problems and loss of libido as a result of testosterone deprivation can all have the effect of releasing the 'demons'.

Over time, other signs and symptoms may manifest, such as:

- feeling deeply sad and hopeless;
- loss of interest in and enjoyment of life and sex;
- difficulty in sleeping or sleeping too much;
- major appetite and weight changes;
- tiredness and loss of energy;
- trouble concentrating;
- feeling helpless or worthless;
- feeling restless, irritable and/or agitated;

- feeling very fragile and on edge; and
- thoughts of suicide or death.

At this stage, if the patient consults a health professional concerning these symptoms, he may be diagnosed as suffering from a degree of reactive depression. Of significance here, following a recent survey from our own Prostate Cancer Support Group in Brisbane, is the fact that more than 50 per cent of men who replied stated they had been diagnosed with or experienced depression.

What to do

It is important to understand that feeling grief or sadness after a major life event is *not* a sign of character weakness; it is normal. However, it is just as important to seek help if these feelings become overwhelming.

Further, feelings of hopelessness and despair can lead to thoughts of suicide and self harm. These thoughts are serious and help *is* available.

Practical suggestions for dealing with depression

Admit your problem and seek help

First, it is important to talk about it: always seek support. Discuss how you feel with a health professional experienced in depression, or someone you feel comfortable with.

Talking is often the first step in managing depression. This alone may be your greatest help. If you prefer anonymity, consider calling the Cancer Helpline (nationwide toll free 131120). Medicines may also be used (these are discussed later).

Admit you may have been affected by what you have been through. What is important, of course, is how you manage this admission. Bad things happen to everybody. Do not waste time trying to apportion blame. Instead of asking 'Why me?', a better question is 'Why not me?'. You are a human being and there are no guarantees in life. It simply happens. There is such a phenomenon in life as luck—good luck and bad luck. Eventually, build bridges, draw a line and put it behind you. Understand what you've been through, accept it, treat it and get on with your life.

Think positive

You cannot afford the indulgence of a negative thought. Such thinking will only reinforce the smoothness of this contrary cerebral pathway, dragging you back into the cauldron. Gather together a whole armament of distractive techniques. Here are a few:

- *Exercise.* Within ten minutes of beginning cardiovascular activity, or exercise, the body releases natural endorphins which often can be enough to neutralise the 'demons'.
- It is often helpful to *visualise* the 'demons' as people— someone you can talk to and control. By sheer will-

power, convince them to go away. (This is similar to what Russell Crowe's character, John Nash, did with his schizophrenic 'demons' in the movie *A Beautiful Mind*).

- Learn to *meditate* or practise a *deep relaxation technique*. This is a highly specific neurological state of the body that requires a specific mental approach. The aim is to abandon one's conscious control and turn over control to the body's in-built 'autopilot'. People who enter this state for fifteen to twenty minutes open their eyes later feeling a sense of peacefulness and release from all previous tension.

- *Stop obsessing.* Give yourself a signal, like snapping a rubber band on your wrist, to vanquish those endlessly negative thoughts.

- *Substitute positive thoughts.* Make yourself think about something wonderful—like planning a holiday, a special creative goal, a present or nice clothes for yourself.

- *Challenge the negative thoughts* by asking: 'Is this really true? Where is the evidence? If my best friend was thinking in this way, what would I tell them?' Be your *own* best friend.

Experience your emotions

Don't suppress or deny any of your feelings. Initially, the idea is to experience the emotions. Learn to recognise them, then learn how to *detach* from them. Learn to talk about your most fearful moments—the worrying times. Maybe your first emotions were shock, fear or anxiety at the time of diagnosis. Maybe when you believed your side-effects were going to last forever, you experienced sadness, rage or great anxiety.

The idea is to recognise the feeling of these emotions, their texture, their moisture, the shiver down the back, the quick flash of heat that crosses your brain—then say: 'OK, this is fear. Step away from it. This is rage. Now forget it.'

Let the emotion wash over you. It won't and can't hurt you. It will only help. If you pull it on like a familiar shirt, then you can say to yourself: 'All right, it's just fear. I don't have to let it control me. I see it for what it is—a primitive reaction—with overkill!'

The same applies to loneliness, sadness and rage. Let the tears flow, feel it completely, but eventually be able to say: 'All right, that was my moment of loneliness. I've felt it and I'm not afraid of it. There are other emotions in the world I want to feel more. I will detach from this.' Send those negative feelings scampering (Albom, 2001).

Medication

Consult your doctor concerning appropriate medication, as some medicines help relieve the symptoms of anxiety. One strategy relates to an attempt to regulate neurotransmitters. Neurotransmitters are chemicals or hormones in the brain which transfer a message across a nerve synapse. Many of these brain chemicals (neurochemicals) have been linked to the development of depression (e.g. norepinephrine, dopamine, serotonin). Stress has been shown to deplete or unbalance these transmitters.

It has been suggested that chronic or severe stress (such as loss of a body function, loss of quality of life, an unexpected medical diagnosis, loss of employment) may cause neurochemical changes therefore triggering episodes of depression.

Antidepressant medicines work to get brain chemicals back in balance. They can help to inhibit certain neurotransmitters that have been associated with the cause of depression. These medicines are not addictive and may help with counselling.

7

Erectile dysfunction: The meaning of manhood

I like to remind patients that cancer is not a vocation. It's not like a job that you've got to get really good at. It's a journey that you have to get through.

—Harvey Max Chuchinov

At a recent prostate cancer support meeting, a particular incident characterised the dilemma often faced by men diagnosed with prostate cancer. One youngish man (in his late forties) was recovering from a prostatectomy. He was fit looking and otherwise appeared to be in good health. However, when he was given an opportunity to speak it became obvious he was seriously distressed.

He said he had been well all his life and was symptom-free at the time of the cancer disclosure. He admitted that he had been dramatically shocked by the diagnosis, to the point that he had become quite angry. As such, he just wanted that 'thing' out of his body as soon as possible—he was prepared to undergo surgery, anything to 'nuke the bastard'.

However, after weathering the radical surgery, he related that he just wasn't prepared for the extent of the emotional trauma he would suffer at the resultant and sudden loss of his erection. Sure, he was warned his erectile function might be compromised, but it hadn't occurred to him the extent to which sex had defined his way of life. Now, he conceded, he was seriously depressed and had even entertained thoughts of suicide. He now regretted his choice of treatment and was after any assistance he could muster.

Immediately, an older man stood up. He'd been there before. With a degree of compassion and obvious understanding he proceeded to reinforce the younger man's earlier decision—that his choice of treatment had been correct and that he should be satisfied with his instincts and initial judgment. He reminded him that he is here now because he chose to narrow the odds of dying young from prostate cancer. This is a trade-off. It looks like a large price to pay now but in the long run it won't be.

And, he continued, it will get easier. He impressed that if he gives it time, he will have sex again, but it will be different. In fact, everything will be different. From the way he approaches most aspects of his life, including his spirituality and how he perceives the purpose and meaning of life, to the relationships with his parents and friends, and certainly how he acknowledges his sex life, it will be different.

The older man continued. He related that when he was undergoing his own treatment he endured many years without sex. 'And,' he said, 'do you know what? Once you've reassessed your life and adapted to the changes, it

really isn't that bad. Give yourself time to come into acceptance and I promise you, your life will be richer in most
aspects.'

The psycho-social aspects

The diagnosis of cancer and what follows have the ability
to dramatically affect your life—to change the way you
view it and the way you live it. It will alter your perspective
on many of life's issues and values, and on many of the
things you once took for granted. If nothing else, it will
force you to confront your mortality and stimulate you to
appreciate and exploit the here and now—this moment—
encouraging you to search for quality of life and whatever
you define happiness to be. With prostate cancer, as well as
the above reactions, it almost certainly will change the way
you view your sexuality and your sex life. Unfortunately,
for some the disease and/or the treatment will seriously
compromise both. However, with insight and patience,
most men will eventually come to the conclusion that the
experience will not be completely to their detriment. Your
life and your sex life *will* be there—it will just be different.

One of the positive effects of a cancer diagnosis is that
it can force you into being more authentic: more aware of
truths and of the fictions of the roles we too easily accept
as our lives. As males, our lives have generally been pro-
grammed on autopilot, fulfilling stereotype and traditional
gender roles placed on us by society. For the most part, we
didn't mind or have any need to question this—the system

worked well, allowing us to gain what we thought was some satisfaction out of life.

That is, until something breaks down—often about mid-life. If, during this breakdown phase, erectile ability is compromised—particularly when it is associated with prostate cancer—then we go into shock and begin to ask questions. Up to this stage, many men probably had adequate functional erections and rarely associated their sex life with their prostate—if, indeed, they even knew what their prostate was. In fact, most men were probably symptom-free prior to treatment, blissfully unaware of any connection between the prostate and sex.

As virtually any form of medical treatment for prostate cancer has the potential to compromise erections and libido, it is no wonder that, when this fate is encountered by a previously sexually active male, a potentially tragic drama begins to unfold. There will be an alarming realisation by the patient of a dampening of the whole delicious anticipatory cycle (diminished reactions to such things as perfumes, or the flash of thigh), leading directly to a potentially negative impact on relationships. Besides dealing with the initial emotional trauma following the diagnosis, a man will quickly suffer a degree of pathos, as he realises he may have lost—probably forever—the central function by which he has previously defined himself as being male.

The fact is, a great many men build their egos and self-esteem around their sex life—often to the point where it could be considered an addiction. This is probably not too harmful in itself, as long as it doesn't lead to unbalanced and anti-social behaviour. Most of the time, we use sex as an obvious reinforcement of our physical expression of our love for our partner. Maybe a couple of times during a lifetime we will use sex to actually have children. The rest of the time it is used for pleasure, a regular thrill, stress relief or a sedative; it can be a creative outlet, something to look forward to or a reward. But, as with all addictions, once the supply is removed, the withdrawal can be painful.

At a time like this, it is important to contemplate some universal truths. What is a male? What is sex? How important is it? Do you really need it? And then deeper ones: What is life? Is there a purpose to it? What about relationships? Happiness? God? . . . and so on.

Adjustment often requires a re-evaluation of values, beliefs, one's faith and the very purpose of being.

In our search for answers, first let's look at the issue of survival.

Survival

In the days immediately following a prostate cancer diagnosis, the issue of survival may overshadow everything else. However, once the crisis subsides, most men hope to resume their previous lifestyle. This is where the problems can start, even though the doctor should certainly have warned the man of the potential side-effects following treatment. When initially balanced against the potential loss of your life, it seems a relatively easy choice to authorise treatment.

Further, the words 'incontinence' and 'impotence' don't really register as important, particularly when mentioned after the word 'cancer' and the phrase 'you could die'. Besides, at this stage most of us probably don't really appreciate the full potential impact of these side-effects. In fairness, probably neither does the doctor, as the chances are he has never experienced them.

Traditional male role

Why do many men place so much emphasis on sex? From a woman's point of view, it would appear we place too much emphasis on it. This difference in perspective, of course, is often a point of tension between partners. Part of the answer can be found by realising that, historically, society's needs have dictated that men fulfil three main roles: the three 'Ps'—that is, Provider, Protector and Procreator (which could also be described as the three 'Ws'—Work, Warrior and Women).

Sex (or procreation) is well known to be one of the strongest male drives. In fact, a recent popular book on the subject has stated that, like it or not, one of the 'ugly' truths about men is that they are thinking about some aspect of sex much of the time, as often as every four minutes, whereas women apparently only think about sex four times a day or less. Further, we realise now that when the prostate gland produces a build-up of seminal fluid, it triggers a mad reflex desire stimulating lustful thoughts about sex. This creates the need to ejaculate and make room for the next lot.

The point is, sex is important to men. However, most of

us take it very much for granted—although we don't realise this truth until it has been taken from us. It is a bit like losing our careers. We become very insecure: we want to feel that we are the providers as well as the procreators.

In fact, most men will become quite angry, not being adequately equipped to emotionally manage the loss. Certainly, most of us will not be aware of the natural stages of grief we may have to pass through after loss—denial, anger and depression—before we come into acceptance.

Are we captive to our manhood?

So, are men held captive in ivory towers of their 'manhood', isolated from emotion, vulnerability and their greater humanity?

At first, it appears that male socialisation supports the case that males' basic experience is the opposite of intimacy. We are not allowed to be seen as vulnerable, to cry or to show weakness of any sort. That is how we define ourselves. After all, our generation was spawned by an unbroken line of men who were imbued with the ideals of chivalry—that is, perfect gentlemen, faithful, courteous to women, pure, brave and fearless, unsparing of self, bowing before God and womenkind—a situation that today is considered by many to be worthy of disdain and largely irrelevant.

The fact is, we've allowed ourselves to believe that aggression is a male trait and vulnerability is a feminine trait. Psychologist Karen Nixon suggests this is wrong. These are not gender roles—they are both human qualities. By accepting this belief, we come to realise that male vulnerability does not disappear; it just becomes unnaturally suppressed, thus rendering us powerless and inexperienced when we are confronted with any threatening condition, such as a disease, job loss or bereavement. We have nowhere to go.

Added to this, society's—and particularly men's—fixation with penetrative sex restricts the whole range of activity which humans crave, such as intimacy and sensual contact. In fact, women universally rate the overall relationship—in terms of warmth, caring, touching and closeness—as being just as important as, if not more so than, erectile function—note that we're talking *sexuality* here, not *sex*. Sexuality relates to being male (or female) and is independent of the ability to have penetrative sex.

A way out?

As tough as it seems, illness can provide us with the capacity to gain some insights and wisdom, to cut through the nonsense and sham concerning our sexuality. Three things have to happen.

First, there is no point in trying to hang on to what you once had. Consider your losses to be a valid trade-off for your life. For most men, however, the losses are not complete. In this case, there are many ways to gain sexual fulfilment—in fact, you need to know that most of you will regain an eminently satisfactory degree of sexual feelings and desire. But it is necessary for couples to work together to accept and embrace the change—to find new opportunities and seek support from family, friends and health professionals. When there is a crisis, there needs to be a sense of the team in a relationship. And it is OK to cry—it is a valid part of the grieving process and a way to cope.

Second, if something happens to your dream, when bad times happen (and they will, because life has no guarantees) don't search for someone or something to blame. You have to stop, take stock, redefine yourself and focus on a new vision.

It may be helpful to understand that the essence of what makes a good man has never changed: trustworthiness, a fierce capacity for love, unselfish action for the common good and the ability to laugh in the face of hardship—no mention of sex here!

Third, if you are left completely impotent—even though most men would rather not have it this way—it is important to realise that the alternative doesn't offer a better scenario: we do not need reminding that 2600 men die of prostate cancer a year in Australia. To cope with the prospects of diminished libido, it is necessary to shift your whole way of thinking. If you give the situation sufficient time and understanding, and if you can persuade yourself to look to the future, you will eventually work through the grief process into a state of acceptance. After all, in the general community, 50 per cent of men over the age of 50 are impotent (from other medical conditions such as diabetes, alcoholism and cardiovascular problems), and this percentage increases by 10 per cent for every decade of life. That means a great many men have been through this and continue to live a meaningful and contented life. You can too.

A word on health professionals

Health professionals must recognise that the diagnosis of prostate cancer can affect the way a man views himself, his sexuality and intimacy for the rest of his life. Coupled with other devastating side effects such as urinary/faecal incontinence and symptoms derived from testosterone deprivation therapies, the overall scenario can quickly force a man into bouts of reactive depression. In fact, research has shown that the worse the impotence, the worse the depression—which can quickly become serious, or even suicidal, if not treated. This aspect of managing prostate cancer has already been shown to be one of the important areas not adequately addressed—one of the 'unmet needs'.

Experience from our support group has shown that some health professionals have trouble initiating a conversation concerning various aspects of these 'unmet needs', particularly sexuality. In fact, this dilemma is probably one of the greatest challenges to many health professionals in their ability to deliver adequate care. Complicating this reticence, of course, is the male patient's unwritten code of silence, intimating 'I'm fine, Doc. Nothing that I can't handle here.'

We would encourage health professionals to be more proactive and use phrases such as:

- How has this treatment affected you sexually?
- How has this experience affected your relationship with your partner or yourself?

- Have you felt down at any stage? Any black days?

Once any problems are uncovered, if the doctor is not confident in personally managing them, he would do his patient a tremendous service to refer him to someone specialising in these issues.

The medical community needs to recognise that treatment of the emotional and psychological side-effects is among the most important issues facing prostate cancer survivors and their families.

Points to ponder

Taking a very different perspective, there may be some who actually welcome this sexual deprivation.

Perhaps we can look at some words of wisdom from the past. In Plato's *Republic*, a man of advanced years described the relief of no longer being obsessed with sex. Many of his fellows, he said, lived in their memories of the pleasures of youth. But not him. He now had time for creative and cerebral outlets.

Nor, apparently, was Sophocles concerned by the impact of advancing age. When the great dramatist was asked whether he still made love to women, he answered: 'Good heavens, no. I have gladly made my escape from that barbarous, savage monster.'

This sentiment is echoed by Cicero and Seneca as they cite various authorities: 'The most fatal curse given to mankind is sensual greed.' 'Age frees us from youth's most dangerous failings.'

These sentiments cannot be taken lightly. One might expect such pronouncements from clerics and individuals who have voluntarily accepted poverty, chastity and obedience, but not from aristocratic geniuses who have tasted the best the ancient world had to offer.

Even though it is easy to suspect that these writings may be a rationalisation of a man making the best of a bad bargain, I believe there may be a message of liberation of sorts if a man can work through his grief into acceptance.

In fact, Ghandi stated that he could never accomplish what he wanted to do unless he could channel the energy which he would normally burn (waste) on his libido and sex drive. He continued by saying that if he could take that energy and direct it in the proper way, he could liberate India. Which he did!

Further, of course, we do have an advantage over the ancients and Ghandi. There are many medical aids that can now assist in attaining an erection. Don't hesitate to consult a doctor with a special interest in male health problems. There is a lot they can do.

However, how we handle erectile dysfunction is ultimately up to us. We have the ability to research and gain information to help ourselves. Perhaps our final comment should come from the chivalrous philosophy of knighthood: 'Once a King, always a King; once a night may be too much.'

Final thought

This quote comes from a leaflet produced by the National Cancer Institute in the United States:

Being a survivor of cancer

Cancer survivorship can be a catalyst for spiritual awakening, providing life and depth and poignancy. Survivors themselves are often gutsy and assertive, and they dare to take chances. They are often optimistic, independent-minded, and compassionate and have elevated self-esteem and pride. New attitudes towards work, pleasure and relationships develop with utmost clarity, while superficial distractions and frivolous people are filtered out . . . [Survivors] share a new understanding of time, and a sense of needing to make every minute count.

Appendix:
Pilot study results

No.	Age	Surgical t'ment	Pre-physio	Physio t'ment	Results post-physio	Remarks
1	69	RAD 10/7/01	6 pads a day 3 pads a night	2/12 post op.	Completely dry by 3/12 post op.	v.v. happy
2	58	RAD Aug/01	4–6 pads a day	3/12 post op.	1/12 after treatment 1–2 pads a day (suggested increase abs → 200 a day) by 2/12 later no pad needed—a little trickle	v. happy (rang 2/12 later almost completely dry)

No.	Age	Surgical t'ment	Pre-physio	Physio t'ment	Results post-physio	Remarks
3	59	RAD 3/9/01	1–2 pads a day	2/12 post op.	By 3/12 after treatment completely dry	v. happy
4	61	RAD 16/10/01	2–3 pads a day	6/52 post op.	1/12 later all dry (did up to 600 abs) few dribbles	v. happy (good abs now also)
5	70	RAD 16/10/01	4 pads a day	7/52 post op.	2/12 later only a small dribble now and then	v. happy
6	71	RAD 2/10/01	Annoying dribble	2/12 post op.	4/12 later dry, except if tired after 18 holes of golf	v. happy
7	58	RAD 7/8/01	1–2 pads a day	4/12 post op.	6/12 later no pads. OK weekends. Loses a few drops at end of work day	v. happy and is going to persist with routine

No.	Age	Surgical t'ment	Pre-physio	Physio t'ment	Results post-physio	Remarks
8	55	RAD 26/11/01	1–2 pads a day	6/52 post op.	6/12 later virtually dry	v. happy
9	69	TURP 20/11/01	1 pad a day	2/12 post op.	3/12 later completely dry	v. happy
10	68	RAD 6/3/02	6 pads a day	6/52	1/12 later down to 2 pads a day. 2/12 later completely dry	thrilled
11	63	RAD 29/11/01	3 pads a day	2/12	1/12 later completely dry	v. happy
12	67	RAD 30/1/02	6–8 pads a day, plus one at night	6/52 post op.	3/12 later completely dry	extremely happy—does 350 sit-ups daily
13	57	RAD 19/4/02	3 pads a day	1/12 post op.	1/12 later completely dry	v. happy

No.	Age	Surgical t'ment	Pre-physio	Physio t'ment	Results post-physio	Remarks
	Av. 63.5		Av. 3.5 pads	Av. 2 months post op.	Av. small dribble only 3 patients after 6 months—other 10 patients dry	

Legend

RAD—radical prostatectomy

TURP—transurethral resection prostate

1/12 = one month, 2/12 = two months, etc.

ABS = abdominal exercises

Bibliography

Albom, Mitch, *Tuesdays with Morrie*, Hodder, Sydney, 2001.

Apell, R., personal communication, Urology Department, Cleveland Clinic, Ohio, 1999.

Chiarelli, Pauline, *Women's Waterworks: Curing Incontinence*, George Parry, Newcastle, NSW, 2002.

Clinical Practice Guideline No. 2, Update: Urinary Incontinence in Adults: Acute and Chronic Management, US Department of Health and Human Services, Maryland, 1996.

Dorey, Grace, *Conservative Treatment of Male Urinary Incontinence and Erectile Dysfunction*, Whurr, London and Philadelphia, 2001.

Hodges, P.W., 'Is there a role for transversus abdominis in lumbo-pelvic stability?' *Manual Therapy* vol. 4, no. 2, 1999, pp. 74–86.

Hodges, P.W. and Richardson, C.A., 'Feed-forward contraction of transversus abdominis is not influenced by the direction of arm movement', *Experimental Brain Research* no. 114, 1997, pp. 362–70.

Mamberti-Dias, A., Vasavada, S.P. and Bourcier, A.P., *Pelvic Floor Dysfunction: Investigations and Conservative Treatment*, Casa Editrice Scientifica Internationale, Paris, 1999, pp. 303–10.

McKenzie, D.K., Gandevia, S.C., Gorman, R.B. and Southon, F.C.G., 'Dynamic changes in the zone of apposition and diaphragm during maximal respiratory effects', *Thorax* no. 49, 1994, pp. 634–8.

Meaglia, J.P., Joseph, A.C., Chang, M. and Schmidt, J.D., 'Post-prostatectomy urinary incontinence: Response to behavioural training', *Journal of Urology* vol. 144, 1990, pp. 674–6.

Men's Health, May 2002, p. 18.

Millard, Richard J., *Bladder Control: A Simple Self-help Guide*, MacLennan & Petty, Sydney, Philadelphia, London, 1996.

Moul, J. W., 'Pelvic muscle rehabilitation in males following prostatectomy', *Urologic Nursing* vol. 18, no. 4, December 1998.

Moul, J.W., Mooneyham, R.D., Kao, T., McLeod, D.G., and Cruess, D.F., 'Preoperative and operative factors to predict incontinence, impotence and stricture after radical prostatectomy', *Prostate Cancer and Prostatic Diseases* vol. 1, no. 5, 1998, pp. 242–9.

Oesterling, J.E. and Moyad, M.A., *The ABCs of Prostate Cancer*, Madison Books, Lanham, New York, Oxford, 1997.

Sapsford, R.R. and Hodges, P.W., 'Contraction of pelvic floor muscles during abdominal manoeuvres', *Archives of Physical Medicine and Rehabilitation* no. 82, 2001, pp. 1081–8.

Sapsford, R.R., Hodges, P.W., Richardson, C.A., Cooper, D.H., Markwell, S.J. and Jull, G.A., 'Co-activation of the abdominal and pelvic floor muscles during voluntary exercises', *Neurology and Urodynamics* no. 20, 2001, pp. 31–42.

Van Kampen, M., De Weerdt, W., Van Poppel, H. et al., 'Effect of pelvic floor re-education on duration and degree of incontinence after radical prostatectomy: A randomized controlled trial', *Lancet* no. 355, 1998, pp. 98–102.

Index